Weight Gain:
When It's Not
Your Fault

Weight Gain:
When It's Not
Your Fault

SIX COMMON MEDICAL CONDITIONS CAUSING WEIGHT
GAIN AND GETTING DOCTORS TO PAY ATTENTION!

Dr. Lance Dean Ashworth

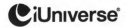

WEIGHT GAIN: WHEN IT'S NOT YOUR FAULT
Six Common Medical Conditions Causing Weight
Gain and Getting Doctors to Pay Attention!

The information, ideas, and suggestions in this book are not intended as a substitute for professional medical advice. Before following any suggestions contained in this book, you should consult your personal physician. Neither the author nor the publisher shall be liable or responsible for any loss or damage allegedly arising as a consequence of your use or application of any information or suggestions in this book.

iUniverse books may be ordered through booksellers or by contacting:

iUniverse
1663 Liberty Drive
Bloomington, IN 47403
www.iuniverse.com
1-800-Authors (1-800-288-4677)

Because of the dynamic nature of the Internet, any web addresses or links contained in this book may have changed since publication and may no longer be valid. The views expressed in this work are solely those of the author and do not necessarily reflect the views of the publisher, and the publisher hereby disclaims any responsibility for them.

Any people depicted in stock imagery provided by Thinkstock are models, and such images are being used for illustrative purposes only. Certain stock imagery © Thinkstock.

ISBN: 978-1-4917-1635-9 (sc)
ISBN: 978-1-4917-1636-6 (hc)
ISBN: 978-1-4917-1637-3 (e)

Library of Congress Control Number: 2013922486

Printed in the United States of America.

iUniverse rev. date: 02/04/2015

CONTENTS

INTRODUCTION

It is official; as of June 2013 the American Medical Association has announced that obesity is a disease. I went to medical school at the Arizona College of Osteopathic Medicine and after completing my post-graduate training in 2002 I opened the first 100% dedicated weight management medicine clinic in Ormond Beach, FL. Even at that early stage of my career I knew obesity was a serious condition that would require all of my training to treat. To be honest it has taken almost all of the last decade to figure out how to properly treat this disease known as Obesity. This is primarily because obesity causes or contributes to a myriad of adverse health conditions, from diabetes and heart disease to high blood pressure and liver abnormalities. The fact that fatty tissue can cause so many health problems is not breaking news though. As early as 400 B.C., Hippocrates wrote, "Sudden death is more common in the naturally fat than in the lean". The breaking news should be that the majority of the medical community I am a part of still does not completely understand the actual pathways that link these disorders together causing the obese condition. This is evident by the purely reactionary approach most of my colleagues take when they are faced with a patient that is obese or clearly on the road to becoming obese. Something needs to change!

This book will show you in easy to understand ways what I meant when I named this book Weight Gain: When It's Not your Fault. Importantly this book will hopefully help you explain to your doctor what it means to be more proactive when treating disorders you may already be suffering from. A perfect example of where a paradigm shift needs to occur is in the treatment of diabetes in the overweight individual. It seems as though my colleagues have been content for years treating the diabetic condition while offering little to no relevant medical advice about weight reduction. In reality, the excess weight was, in all likelihood, the cause of their diabetic condition in the first place. It is no surprise that the steadily rising number of individuals suffering with obesity is only matched by the steadily rising number of type II diabetics. If you are overweight and are worried about having diabetes I will show you a much more effective way to approach the diagnosis of diabetes years before your sugar levels begin to rise. Because once those sugar levels rise you have already damaged your body.

This book has been written by a weight management medicine doctor in an effort to help *you* help *your* doctors diagnose and treat the root causes of weight gain; this book will help you increase the length and quality of your life. When you treat the correct medical problem, reducing weight and then maintaining the weight lost occurs much easier. This book will give you the information you need to encourage your doctor to take a more aggressive, proactive approach in helping you reduce your weight. *Until the correct medical problem has been addressed by your doctor, gaining weight and subsequently not being able to lose it is not your fault.*

Let me put it another way. If you are diagnosed with a disease too late and then treated improperly and this disease begins to affect other organ systems causing further complications, most people would agree that it was not your fault. But although most federal agencies, many insurance companies, and now the AMA agree that obesity is a full-blown disease process, if you show up at your doctor's office for a checkup and the only problem is a steady weight gain, most physicians will not diagnose you with a disease. Obesity has the potential to be the direct cause of diabetes and a multitude of various cancers and can cause the heart to drastically increase in size, to name but a few of the resultant medical issues that arise secondarily to the disease obesity. Yet the medical establishment's attitude towards this disease in the early stages is pathetically lackadaisical.

As a person grows in size the medical problems that arise as a direct result of this overabundance of fatty tissue are so numerous it makes the head spin. These conditions are not harmless; on the contrary they are without a doubt life threatening. By the time attention is drawn to the obese condition it is usually only because the patient now has Type II Diabetes, High Blood Pressure, or Sleep Apnea; in other words, a tangible disease that the doctor is able to place in a neat package and write a prescription for. These medical problems are in most cases secondary to the weight gain that should have been diagnosed as obesity and aggressively treated years before. The diagnosis of obesity with all of the associated diseases that stem from it are as lethal as cancer. Not to mention that obesity can also lead to cancer.

In the pages that follow I will go through many of the most common disorders that need to be tested for, diagnosed, and most importantly treated properly and in a timely manner when you find yourself gaining weight. The conditions I write about in this book are those that commonly cause abnormal weight gain or are the direct result of weight gain. A large percent of my patients assume their doctors are testing and treating these conditions properly. They most assuredly are not. If they were, the percent of people in this country suffering with or on their way to becoming obese would not be on the rise. So many people are burdened by obesity because it is multi-faceted in its causes and treatment options.

Obesity is so prevalent in our society because in order to address this condition doctors need to consider the medical, genetic, social, emotional, and cultural relationships. But compared to other prevalent conditions such as severe depression, the amount of resources and research dedicated to finding the causes and treatment options for obesity is inadequate. When seeking obesity treatments by your doctor, all of the above issues mentioned at the beginning of this paragraph needs to be addressed. I believe the reason so many people are overweight is because so few doctors are willing or have the time and resources to deal with all of those issues. Working in weight management medicine throughout the years has taught me that contrary to popular belief, <u>not everyone who is overweight simply eats too much and refuses to exercise.</u>

Throughout this book you will find testimonials from my past patients. I placed them in the book in the hopes that some of what they say may ring true in your own life. This book will address many of the medical and non-medical concerns, which in my experience will help to ensure success in reducing weight and keeping it off. In addition to the medical concerns that need to be addressed, a major area of concern is teaching you how to eat properly. The glycemic index (GI) of foods has major implications for the prevention and treatment of sickness and death associated with obesity in the US. The glycemic index measures how quickly a food is digested. Therefore it represents how that food affects the subsequent response of sugar and insulin. I cannot stress how important controlling insulin is when attempting to reduce weight.

As a physician in the practice of weight management medicine, I strive to cure the conditions caused by obesity. Conditions many of my physician colleagues seem content in simply slowing in progression. I am often asked why I chose to focus on obesity as a physician. Aside from the obvious medically based answer provided in the previous sentence, there is a more personal reason. Helping people reduce weight and being given the opportunity to motivate them is an honor and a privilege for me. I am passionate about what I do, and patients can feel that I genuinely want to help them change their life. Building a level of mutual trust and respect is crucial. After diagnosing what is wrong medically with their weight gain issues, the majority of my time is spent talking with my patients each week. Every patient comes to understand that I truly want to find the underlying medical and psychological reasons behind their weight issues.

Sometimes I feel like I am living the life of Riley, having the chance to do exactly what I want in life. Patients feel my sincerity when we are trying to get to the bottom of a psychological issue that has been bothering them. They do not feel as though they are taking too long, or taking up the doctors' precious time. With new people who come to see me I walk into the room and look at a man or woman that may weigh exceedingly more than their *ideal weight* and they see that I am looking at them. I look into their eyes and start the process of figuring out who they are as a person, not a chart, not a number, but a person that needs me. This sort of personal one on one attention is something many overweight individuals are not accustomed to. The sad part is that this is not my personal opinion, but a situation that has been recited to me time and time again by my patients. Overweight or obese individuals are looked over, looked through and ignored, not only in public but in many cases right in the doctors' office. Regardless of how tired I am at the end of the day, being in the room and starting to talk about a patient's journey towards health rejuvenates my mind and spirit. This in turn transforms a timid, nervous patient into someone who is equally rejuvenated and excited about the journey. It should be easy to understand why I love what I do and why I chose this area of medicine.

Why read this book? My wife was one of the first people to read this book while it was still on the computer. She commented that if she were to pick just one word to describe what this book offered, it would be empowerment. Knowledge is power. Knowledge is even more important in the medical community where acquiring and retaining knowledge is all that separates a highly qualified doctor from a mediocre one. Aside from that elusive quality called common sense. Having common sense allows doctors to understand that thinking outside of the typical medical box opens up a world of possibilities that others may not have considered. Doctors with common sense keep their mouth shut and let their patients do the talking. When this occurs the patient will usually tell the doctor enough to make the diagnosis easier. If you are lucky enough to find a doctor with common sense that allows you to talk, it would be beneficial as well to have been empowered by this book as my wife mentioned. Look at what you are about to read as a guide book written for you, a person that is ready to lead their doctor down a path that doctor may have otherwise been unaware of.

The medical environment as previously stated is way too reactionary. When I was asked to give one word that I hoped this book would accomplish, it was a word I would apply to both the reader and their doctors: proactive. In the treatment of obese patients a proactive physician would need to adopt an almost complete change in standard of care. Over the years it has seemed as if physicians have become progressively more reactionary and content to only treat what is staring them in the face. This is most evident when looking at the diagnosis and treatment of diabetes in overweight individuals. We have tried just about everything to get control of diabetes. Common sense dictates that if what we have been doing is not working it is time to try a different approach. With diabetes continually on the increase a paradigm shift is in order as far as I am concerned. I can only hope that it will start with you the reader, the patient and your influence on your personal physician.

When my patients have described the weight management advice they have received, or lack thereof from other so called weight loss programs, I knew a book like this had to be written. Weight management is hard enough when everything is in order. Trying to get it done with bad advice or no advice from medical professionals is unacceptable and unsuccessful. It can be very shocking to find out that the weight you have been carrying around for so long could have been made easier to lose if a hormone or medication was addressed in the past. Keep in mind that the information in this book is not coming from a lay person without any experience treating patients, who claims to know what they are talking about because they have read all of the research. This book was hammered out by a doctor practicing weight management medicine. It is coming from a doctor who has trampled down the resistance, ignored the ridicule, and spent the last decade creating the path you can lead your doctor down. Read the book, learn what treatment you need and deserve, and go get it!

Throughout the book you will find what we call in medicine "Pearls", or in this case "Pearls of Wisdom" or POW's. These are simply small reminders of the more important details I do not want forgotten from that particular topic. These POW's will also keep you from continuing to be a POW (Prisoner of your Weight).

CHAPTER 1

What to Look for in a Weight Management Doctor

I wrote this section to primarily make the reader aware of what to look for when attempting to find a weight management medicine doctor. When I was in my residency, more than a couple of my supervisors told me I was crazy to open up a clinic dedicated 100 percent to weight management medicine. One or two of them had tried to add weight management to their clinics and were unsuccessful. Of course, upon further questioning it became evident that the "weight loss clinics" they had opened were little more than giving the patient a reduced calorie program and an appetite suppressant. If the patient was experiencing low and slow weight loss the answer was to exercise more and eat less. Did these doctors attempt to find an underlying cause for the weight gain? If they had I would not have felt the need to write this book, and they might have actually had a successful weight management clinic.

Their prediction was that I would be out of business in less than two years. They said I was competing against the commercial weight management centers that had deep pockets for advertising. I told them I had no competition because there was only one "me" out there. Unless those commercial weight management centers were planning on cloning me, I felt as though no one was doing weight management the way I felt it should be done. After over a decade, I have proved all of them wrong. Not to say there have not been ups and downs. But in my community I have always been the physician to come see for fast, safe weight management as well as Bio-Identical Hormone Replacement Therapy.

In Florida, I spent most of my career on the East coast of the state and after around five years I felt as though if I could make it work there I could make it work in other places. I opened up additional clinics in the state. I hired and trained Nurse Practitioners that could render the type of care that needed to be given. I basically duplicated the program I created on the east coast of Florida. The only difference was that it was not going to be me that the patient would see each time they came in. The majority of the time it would be a nurse practitioner that the patient would see. After a year and a half I decided to close these clinics. The patients just did not seem to do as well as they had in the past. The patient and doctor referrals for the programs were not what they should have been as compared to the original east coast location; where I was seeing patients on a regular basis using the same programs that were being offered at the other clinics. For the life of me, I could not figure out how to make those other clinics work.

It became apparent that what I did when I was the one seeing my patients was intangible and difficult, if not impossible to duplicate. Not to mention the fact that when the patient reads the clinic is owned by *Dr. Lance Ashworth* they wanted to see Dr. Ashworth, not a different doctor, a nurse practitioner, or a physician's assistant. This is not to say that these types of practitioners could not be successful. What it does say is that doing weight management part-time or allocating the patient contact to someone else may be what prevents the patients from being successful. There is an element of expectation present when a person walks in the door of a weight management medicine clinic.

If a clinic is not successful it may be that the doctor is attempting to see the weight management patients in the same way they see their regular internal medicine or family practice patients. The name of the game these days in a managed care environment and a tough economy is how many patients can the doctor see in an hour? This will not work in weight management medicine. Patients in a weight management program need extra time to simply talk about how they felt that week. This may be how they felt mentally instead of strictly physically. There may be nothing to actually *treat* in the strict sense of the word at that particular visit. The patient may simply need a motivational, hunger, or exercise tip.

Patients who are seeing someone for weight management expect to be motivated long after any diagnoses related to gaining weight have been diagnosed and treatment began. It seems that patients can feel when a doctor really cares about them and why that doctor is sitting in front of them. Attempting to cram these patients through the door and see as many as possible will not be successful for very long. My patients get to know me as well as I know them. I became acutely aware of this when patients would ask me what was wrong or why I looked so stressed out. A strong relationship of trust and mutual respect needs to be developed. It is as if the patient should want to lose weight for all the correct medical and personal reasons, but also for the doctor. Being capable of fostering this type of relationship is difficult to teach a doctor, they either can do it or they cannot. Motivating patients, putting them at ease, or relieving their stress is something that comes natural to a physician or it does not.

The amazing part of all of this is that the patients can feel it. I believe it is because they have usually been through a lot. By that I mean everything from multiple programs and treatment styles, to straight out abuse from the people around them. Sadly, the worst abuse is often from those closest to them, like their husband, wife, or parents. They have been ignored, thought of as lazy, physically abused, and in the process have had their self-confidence destroyed. It takes a certain type of doctor to be able to relate to these patients and earn their trust. That is what I tell every patient. I am their personal weight management doctor and we are a team.

I put this in the book for you, the reader, to help you find a doctor that will help you lose weight. When this may be your "last-ditch effort", it needs to be the correct type of health practitioner. They will either be cut out for the job or not. A lot of that is dependent on their personality. A lot depends on their ability to be able to treat each patient differently according to their needs. It takes a bit of common sense. There is no cookie cutter way of doing weight management. The future of medical weight management, the paradigm shift I would like to see is one where every patient is looked at as a whole: the entire array of symptoms, the patient's personality, and lab results need to come together as a whole. Nothing is taken alone and looked at individually to direct an entire treatment protocol. The future of weight management medicine is figuring out why the patient gained the weight, not just treating the diseases the excess weight is causing. Physicians need to come out of the safety of the "medical box" and treat underlying disorders that may be making weight management impossible. As you read through the different disorders think about how you feel, the medications you take, and attempt to find yourself in these pages. Be prepared to take what you learn and share the information with your doctor. There is treatment available. Being overweight or obese is not a death sentence or a lifelong condition. Knowledge is power. Unfortunately common sense is not that common in the medical community. Read on and let the knowledge empower you to help your doctor help you.

POW: **THE MOST IMPORTANT PART TO LOOK FOR IN A WEIGHT MANAGEMENT PROGRAM OR PROVIDER IS THEIR FOCUS ON FIGURING OUT WHY YOU GAINED THE WEIGHT FROM A *MEDICAL STANDPOINT.***

CHAPTER 2

What to Look for at your First Visit

Before jumping right in, I thought it would be a good idea to go through a typical *Initial Consult*. I am including this because of the sheer number of so called "physician managed weight loss clinics" people are exposed to. This book helps you understand what to look for when a doctor or even a commercial weight management center gets you into the consultation room or "hot seat," whichever applies, and begins to talk about how they will help you lose weight. There are certain subjects and key words that these people should mention, or questions that need to be asked of you that will be the signal that you are in the right place. I also suggest questions that you can ask that will validate that you are in the right place. Go in with confidence. They are lucky to have you in their establishment. You put them on the hot seat and see if they truly know what they are doing.

Right from the start I must say that I never try to talk anyone into starting my weight management program. I simply present what I am able to do and see if the patient and I are compatible. You should not feel pressure or feel like you are being subjected to tactics to get you to start a weight management program. As a matter of fact, I have flat-out told people they are not ready and told them to return when they are absolutely sick of being overweight. I tell them this because if they are a little bit "ok" being overweight, when the rubber meets the road and the newness of the weight management program wears off, they will feel a whole lot more "ok" being overweight. Just like I tell you that there are certain words you need to be looking for, I also look for certain people when they enter my clinic. I try to determine if this is going to be a person that is going to give it their all or someone who is going to give up when the going gets tough.

One of the major obstacles the general public perceives when they think about seeing a doctor for weight management is the money needed to get the job done. The reality is that people end up *saving* money when they are on a low calorie or very low calorie program. When one looks at the economic environment we are in it is especially important to address the misconception that reducing weight is expensive. The USDA has done many studies looking at the cost of food and the cost of food while on a weight management program and utilizing medically manufactured shakes to supplement nutrition. When the USDA has taken into account the food bought for in home consumption as well as eating out, the results have consistently shown that the person actually saves money while reducing weight and becoming healthier. This is not rocket science and I feel as though if a person really wants to lose weight they will come in having done the math and should be ready to start the process of getting healthy.

If you feel like you are walking into a weight loss clinic with the feel of a gym or fitness center type of atmosphere where high pressure sales tactics are being used just walk out. Or better yet turn the tables and ask them a question: "I'm really feeling pressured to start treatment here and it makes me feel uncomfortable, are you trying to make me feel this way?" Do not let anyone pressure you into starting a weight management program. You will know if a clinic feels right. Go with your gut feeling.

I have never used contracts that lock a person into paying a certain amount over a period of time. Patients pay for a month of weight management at the beginning of each month. If a patient finishes a month and still needs to lose more weight, then they will pay for another month. If something occurs in their life or the person just loses the will to continue the weight management program, I refund the amount paid for the month less any services or products received by the patient. There is no magic wand that will make a person stick to a weight management program. If a clinic or fitness center attempts to lock you into a contract over a specified length of time, run. They should not need a contract. If they are successful at helping people lose weight they should not require a contract to keep you in the program. Most importantly, it is vital to have a medical professional treating you. Avoid the programs that are **approved** by doctors or **created by doctors**. You do not want an establishment where you never see these elusive doctors. Most of these places change management and front office staff like the changing of the weather. They have you take a handful of pills and give you a diet they copied out of some physician's or dietitian's book that is supposed to apply to EVERYONE.

Before everyone out there with a degree other that of an MD or DO gets all bent out of shape let me explain myself. Professionals with these degrees have the training, experience and responsibility to know which symptoms, physical exam findings and lab tests to perform and subsequently interpret that will enable a timely diagnosis as to why the patient gains weight so easily. A question you should feel comfortable asking, and one that should apply to any weight management medicine program is: "What is it that makes your program successful in helping people lose weight?" With the large numbers of individuals in this country being overweight, if a clinic is successful you should have heard about it if the doctor has been around over five years. Most of my patients are word of mouth referrals from previous patients. Before seeing me the patient fills out a questionnaire that I look at which lists their medicines and health conditions and includes many questions on eating and exercise patterns. Everyone is different and requires discussions of different topics and issues. When deciding on a primary care doctor it is very important to find one that is proactive in terms of their patient's weight and body fat percent. Doctors understand, or should understand that gaining weight can cause diabetes. When a trend of weight gain begins, the doctor should focus on the weight. Focusing on the weight is not simply telling the person to stop eating so much, exercise more, and proceeding to write a prescription appetite suppressant medication. So if this is not how a weight management program should start then what is, you may ask an appropriate starting point?

I have always strongly believed that any good first step is for the doctor to order some blood work. Some of the blood work I typically order is not in the standard lab profile, but I am alarmed that some of the common lab work I require has recently been dismissed and removed as necessary in making crucial diagnoses. The treatment of conditions such as Type II Diabetes and Hypothyroidism absolutely require common sense! With obesity causing so many diseases it should be no surprise that I consider all aspects of a person's health profile critical. The doctor needs to take the medical history, the physical exam, the labs and everything else that goes into uncovering a diagnosis. A doctor should never depend on one lab value and make any determination of a person's health without taking all that has been mentioned above into consideration also. This type of medicine, where we look at the person as a whole is starting to be referred to as "Functional Medicine". A doctor needs to be ready to spend 30 to 45 minutes at an initial consult making sure the patient feels comfortable and trusts the doctor. If this doctor is not their primary care doctor it is probably just another program of many the patient has tried and they are more than just a little skeptical. It is our jobs as weight management medicine doctors to put this skepticism to rest, to put you at ease and assure you that you are in the right place.

Laboratory Test Guide

Since one of the goals of this book is to teach the reader what to ask of their doctor, I feel it necessary to give a brief explanation of what some of the more common lab tests really mean in laymen's terms. In order to discover what may be at fault for your weight gain the best place to start is to help you understand the labs that uncover these six disorders. The best way to use these terms would be to have a copy of your lab work in front of you prior to leaving for your doctor's office and go down the list looking for explanations of the results that are of interest. *You will learn what is of interest and what disorders apply to you by the end of this book.* Something worth mentioning is that the values below are not a complete list. Not to worry though, I describe many of the other pertinent labs as I write about the disorders later on in the book. The bold print is how the lab will be written on your lab results.

- **Glucose** is the main source of energy for living organisms. The most important cause of an elevated fasting value is diabetes, but many other factors can also elevate glucose in the blood and urine. Even more important is to know that once this level is high when you haven't eaten in 12 hours, you have had diabetes for a long time. In other words there is a different test that should be looked at when a doctor is initially looking for diabetes and that is an insulin level. Not to worry, this is explained in the diabetes section.

- **Hemoglobin A1C** tests are used to measure diabetes control over a 4 month period (basically the life time of a red blood cell). When elevated it is a sign of poor overall control of the body's sugar levels.

- **Creatinine** is a waste product released from tissue and is excreted from the kidneys. It can become elevated as diabetes or high blood pressure remains uncontrolled and damages the kidneys.

- **Alkaline Phosphatase** is an enzyme found primarily in the liver and bones. Elevated levels may indicate the presence of bone or a variety of liver disorders.

- **Total Bilirubin** levels that are abnormally high may occur in individuals with liver and gall bladder diseases which at times produce jaundice (a yellow discoloration of the skin).

- ***AST or SGOT** is an enzyme found in muscle, heart, and liver cells. Elevated levels can indicate liver and muscle disorders. In people that drink a lot of alcohol this enzyme may go up with liver damage.

- ***ALT or SGPT** is also an enzyme found in muscle, heart, and liver cells. Elevated levels are more often associated with viral disorders of the liver rather than alcohol consumption. This enzyme is also a measure of the degree of damage to the liver.

- ***GGT or GGTP** is a liver enzyme. Unlike other liver enzymes this one is more directly related to alcohol consumption and the resulting damage. This enzyme can also elevate from damage to the liver caused by intake of medications.

  *As a side note, it is normal for the above three liver enzymes to raise and lower during active weight management.

- **Total Protein** in the blood includes two major components, albumin and globulin. Having your protein in balance is important when trying to lose weight. Obviously too little protein in the body will hinder the ability to build muscle, and too much can damage the kidneys.

  o **Albumin** is the largest portion of total blood protein. Decreased levels can indicate many diseases, including advanced liver disease.

  o **Globulin** is a major component of blood proteins. It has many functions including maintenance of the immune system. Elevated and decreased levels may indicate infections, allergic states, immune disorders and other diseases.

- **Total Cholesterol** is a primary risk factor for heart disease which can be controlled. High levels are associated with blocked arteries and heart attacks.

- **HDL** protects against heart disease by picking up bad cholesterol and carrying it back to the liver to be processed for excretion. It is also interesting to note that if the level is markedly elevated it may indicate heavy alcohol intake.

- **LDL** is another marker used to determine the risk of heart disease. The higher the level, the higher the risk of heart disease.

- **Triglycerides** are fats that provide a major reserve of energy for the body. Increases in these as well as other fats are predictors of heart disease.

- **Total Cholesterol/HDL Ratio** is a predictor of heart disease risk. A ratio of less than 4.5 is associated with a lower risk.

- **LDL/HDL Ratio** is calculated using total cholesterol, HDL, and triglycerides. The lower the ratio the less risk of heart problems.

- **Prostate Specific Antigen (PSA)** testing in males has become a bit controversial, but this test is still used as a screening to detect prostate cancer as well as benign enlargement of the prostate. Early detection of prostate cancer is the key to a cure because the disease is usually clinically silent until it has spread.

- **Vitamin D3** or cholcalciferol has been found to play a role in the process of reducing weight. It is actually a pro-hormone and helps with the absorption of calcium and strengthens the immune system.

> _POW:_ _DEMAND THE LABS YOU NEED, DO NOT TAKE NO FOR AN_
> _ANSWER.I WILL GIVE YOU THE LABS YOU NEED, AND YOU MAKE_
> _SURE YOUR DOCTOR ORDERS THEM_

We will now focus on what a work-up should look like for a menopausal woman with a long history of not being able to lose weight. One of a doctor's first duties is to classify each patient, male or female as to the amount of weight they carry, and which diseases they are most at risk for developing based on their body mass index.

Figure 1: Patient classification using their BMI		
Category	BMI (Body Mass Index)kg/m2	Risk of developing other diseases
Underweight	< 18.5	Low
Normal range	18.5-24.9	Average
Overweight	25.0-29.9	Mildly Increased
Obese	>or= 30.0	
Class I	30.0-34.9	Moderate
Class II	35.0-39.9	Severe
Class III	>or= 40.0	Very severe

This table is only meant to put patients in a general classification during the initial work-up. The BMI only takes into account weight and height. Because of the inherent limitations of using only two parameters the table can be taken the wrong way. One of the main reasons is because there is no differentiation between weight that is lean muscle and weight that is fatty tissue. When the press came out a few years ago and said that certain movie stars or athletes were obese it disgusted me. These people had large amounts of lean muscle and were not tall enough to offset that weight. They were in no way, shape, or form obese. They just had a lot of lean muscle which is heavier than fat. This did not do the obese population any favors. It probably did a lot of damage. I could just imagine these people looking at those particular movie stars and thinking if they are obese and look like THAT there is definitely no hope for me. The fact is muscle does weigh more than fat! It is ludicrous to say "A **pound** of muscle weighs the same as a **pound** of fat" Of course it does, just like a pound of feathers weighs the same as a pound of muscle! Because a pound is well . . . a pound! To help you visualize how ridiculous it is to say anything else just read on. If you took a pound of fat and a pound of lean muscle would each of them fit into the same size container? NO, they would not. The container having the pound of fat would be much larger than the container that had a pound of muscle. The more important point is that we are referring to a human being, a body that has a limited amount of space depending on which part of the body we are referring to. If we say that a person's legs are a certain size and we then scrutinize these legs as to what they contain, muscle or fat, if you fill that space with <u>muscle as opposed to fat</u> <u>those legs will weigh MORE!</u> This is why two women can weigh the same but the woman with the larger percent of muscle will have a lower body fat percent, can fit into smaller clothes, and would not necessarily need to lose weight. The other woman may have a higher body fat percent and need to lose weight, <u>yet they weigh the</u> <u>same</u>. We need to break loose from the dramatic and concentrate on the problem: Is it fat we are dealing with, and if so, why does this person gain it so easily? It may not be as popular in the media but at least it will be the truth.

Figure 2: An appropriate, basic weight management medicine workup
<u>Medical History</u>: Careful review of patient's medical history and prescription medications.
<u>Vitals & EKG</u>: Patient's vitals, including weight, blood pressure, pulse, and waist measurement at belly button.
<u>Resting Metabolic Rate</u>: Knowing your *resting metabolic rate* is something I consider basic and required. If a weight management clinic does not measure this, I would consider the program inferior.
<u>Complete Physical Exam</u>: It is vital that I make sure you are not going to hurt yourself when you are exercising. Testing the strength of your muscle and tendon response is part of each exam, as well as listening to your heart and lungs and the other basics of a good physical.
<u>Labs</u>: Order Labs that are relevant to the patient's condition and medical history. The usual labs that are ordered for all patients are a <u>complete</u> <u>metabolic panel</u> that looks at electrolytes, kidneys, and liver function etc. <u>Thyroid studies</u> to include: TSH, T3, T4, and a <u>CBC</u> that helps to look at a patient's red blood cells and possible anemia. Vitamin D3, which is actually a pro-hormone, and lastly a <u>Cholesterol Panel</u>. These are the **basic** labs that are drawn on every patient. If a patient is post-menopausal or exhibiting signs of low testosterone, or other disease processes are suspected such as diabetes additional hormone labs will be requested.

Program Expectations: Once we are done and about to start going over the program I tell every patient there is only three things they must do for me. Drink 64 ounces of "at rest" water, exercise for a minimum of 30 minutes 4 out of 7 days, and do their best to stay on the food program. There is only one that must be attempted perfectly . . . drinking the water. Most of my patients will falter on the other two, but the water intake needs to be near perfect. Trying to be a perfectionist in the other two categories will only lead to frustration.

PATIENT TESTIMONIAL:

Dear Dr. Ashworth,

I was so miserable & self-conscience because of my weight, which was 269 Lbs and I am 6'1" tall. I was huge and couldn't even look at myself in the mirror. I became desperate and knew I needed to do something fast! I looked into vitamins and over the counter diet pills. I've read the possible side effects such as loose bowels, constipation, upset stomach etc. On Dr. Ashworth's weight management program I did not need to take a handful of pills and didn't experience any of these.

I was hoping Dr. Ashworth had a magic wand to make the weight disappear. He didn't but as the days flew by, the pounds did seem to vanish. My diet consisted of a combination of low calorie and low glycemic level foods, increased water intake, and just a couple of protein shakes to help stave off the hunger and help with exercise. After a year, I started to take a prescription appetite suppressant which allowed me to continue to lose weight without the increasing hunger.

With Doctor Ashworth's time, trust, and his suggestions I became a new woman with a new life style and much better self esteem! I lost a total weight of another person . . . . 115 lbs. It was a steady loss of 2 pounds per week (sometimes more, depending on my exercise), which Dr. Ashworth assured me was the best way to lose the weight and keep it off because we were not able to drop the calorie count too low with just two shakes on board.

I look forward to resuming Saturday mornings in the park with Dr. Ashworth during his "walk with the Doc" program whereby he instills in us a healthy way of life.

CS, Florida

> *POW: MUSCLE IS BOTH HEAVIER THAN FAT AND MORE METABOLICALLY ACTIVE THAN FAT. TO INCREASE YOUR METABOLIC RATE, INCREASE YOUR AMOUNT OF MUSCLE.*

CHAPTER 3

Are your Medications causing your Weight Gain?

As a first step every physician should take a hard look at what medications each person takes. It does not matter what the patient may be coming in to see them for on a given day, all of the medications taken on a daily basis should be reviewed for any changes that have been made. In many cases there may be changes that were not advocated under specific medical advice, but on the advice of a well meaning relative or website. More to the point of this book the medication list may unveil a perfect place to start on the journey towards a more healthy weight and lifestyle. In this section I will briefly mention a few of the more common medications that have been found to have a negative effect on a patients' efforts to lose weight or a drug may be the culprit in a patients initial weight gain.

Anticonvulsants:

Tegretol, Neurontin, Lyrica, and Depakote can actually stimulate the production of fat, inhibit the breakdown of fat, and cause water retention. Neurontins' weight gain is dose related in many individuals, the higher the dose of the medicine the more weight that is gained. Lithium blocks dopamine receptors, which leads to increased appetite. *Lithium can also inhibit thyroid hormone synthesis leading to a decreased metabolic rate!*

Antidepressants/Mood Stabilizers:

Antidepressants in the MAO Inhibitor class, such as Nardil, are known to cause weight gain. Remeron blocks histamine, serotonin, and alpha-1 receptors, which leads to increased appetite. SSRI's, most notably Paxil, showed that 25.5% of patients had 7% or greater increase in body weight. These Selective Serotonin Reuptake Inhibitors are more likely to have the weight gain over the long term, as opposed to short-term therapy. Increased appetite and carbohydrate cravings occur with Prozac, Celexa, and Zoloft. Lithium blocks dopamine receptors, but what you need to know is that this can lead to increased appetite. This drug also inhibits thyroid hormone synthesis leading to a decreased metabolic rate!

Antipsychotics:

These can cause increased appetite through serotonin and dopamine receptor blockade. If the medicine also blocks histamine receptors, the patient will experience sedation and decreased physical activity. The worst offender is Clozaril, followed by Seroquel and Risperdal.

Antihistamines:

These can cause weight gain through an increase in appetite when they block histamine H1 receptors. Medicines in this class are Zyrtec, Benadryl, Allegra, and Vistaril. Claritin has shown no data suggesting it causes weight gain.

High Blood Pressure Medications:

These medicines with blockade of peripheral alpha-receptors, such as Minipress and Hytrin, cause weight gain through increased appetite. Beta-blockers, like Tenormin and Inderal, while causing fatigue in many people also decrease metabolic rate, increase insulin resistance, and decrease the breakdown of fat causing weight gain. Centrally acting (working at the level of the brain) medications, like Catapres and Aldomet, which act on the brain stem to stimulate alpha-2-receptors increase appetite leading to weight gain. The medicine Loniten (Minoxidil) causes weight gain primarily through water retention.

Diabetic Medications:

The medication Avandia can cause increased appetite, increased fat storage, and water retention. These other offenders cause an increase in insulin secretion (insulin is absolutely the last hormone we want to be increasing when attempting to lose weight), like Glucotrol. If Glucotrol's problem is an increase in insulin it stands to reason that using insulin in the form of an injection would be a bigger problem. This is indeed the case and the reason why the first goal of any weight management doctor who is treating a Type II diabetic on insulin is to begin decreasing the daily dose of insulin injected from day one. It is truly amazing how much easier reducing weight becomes as the daily dose of insulin is lowered. When on a weight reduction program the body's need for insulin lowers with the lowered amount of food intake, the reduced amount of carbohydrates (sugar) in those reduced calorie portions, as well as the reduction in overall fat the body experiences with weight reduction in general, which decreases insulin resistance. Attempting to lose weight without adjusting diabetic medications can not only make weight reduction a nightmare, but can be life threatening as well. This is explained in more detail in the chapter that covers diabetes.

This is just another of the many reasons why it is so important to have a qualified physician managing your weight reduction. Only a licensed physician can change, adjust or stop any of the medications listed above. Weight management can be nearly impossible if some of the medicines listed are not prescribed with an eye on how they may affect your ability to lose weight. At times, a single medication adjustment can mean the difference between failing and succeeding. This poses a significant problem in this country with so few doctors willing to practice weight management, and so many commercial weight loss centers that have no medical guidance. However, it does not matter how badly you may feel a medication listed above is affecting your weight gain; never discontinue, increase, or decrease any medication listed in this book without the advice of a licensed physician.

POW: **IT IS VITAL TO ADDRESS ALL OF THE MEDICATIONS YOU TAKE, SINCE THE ONLY ONE QUALIFIED TO DO SO IS A DOCTOR, IT MAKES SENSE TO FIND ONE TO HELP YOU REDUCE YOUR WEIGHT.**

CHAPTER 4

Diabetes: The most pervasive
of these disorders

Diabetes is the ultimate enemy to reducing weight. It is estimated that over 8 million people in the U.S. are unaware that they have diabetes! Heart disease is the leading cause of diabetes related deaths. There is a 2-4 fold higher heart disease-related death rate than adults without diabetes. There is also evidence that retinopathy, a disease that can cause blindness, has a chance to worsen over the course of **7 years before the diagnosis of diabetes is even made.**

The hormone, insulin, begins to rear its ugly head even before you have gotten to the point where you begin to think, "Wow, I've really got to get this weight off". Most people refuse to accept the possibility that they are diabetic until their blood sugar levels are high. A lot of patients come to me with a diagnosis of being "pre-diabetic". The truth is that they have been under the solid diagnosis of being a diabetic for probably 5 years. Their insulin levels, **not the sugar levels** have most likely been elevated for at least this long in a futile effort by the pancreas (the gland that makes insulin)to keep those blood sugars normal. The problem is that the pancreas begins to wear out and gets overwhelmed after a few years of pumping out so much insulin and basically being ignored. This is when the blood sugars begin to rise. That is when the dreaded diagnosis of "You've got Type 2 Diabetes" is made. The pancreas has worn out and cannot keep the sugars down any longer, and you finally get the diagnosis that should have been made years before. It could have been made years before by simply measuring the fasting insulin levels. Or at the very least made the correlation that as the patients weight crept up so did the fasting sugars, even if every time they were measured the level was normal. It's called being a little more proactive, watching for trends in the labs; or understanding in one's medical treatment that as a person gains weight, especially around the midsection that this may render that person insulin resistant.

Figure 3: Major Risk Factors for Developing Type II Diabetes

Family History

Obesity (>120% over desired weight or BMI >= 27)

Race/Ethnicity (e.g., Black, Hispanic, Native American, Pacific Islander)

Age >= 45 years old

Had a previous increased fasting sugar test, or increased insulin test

High Blood Pressure = >140/90 mm/Hg

HDL (the good cholesterol) <35 and/or Triglycerides >250

History of gestational diabetes mellitus (sugar goes up in the "mother to be" during pregnancy) or delivery of babies >9 lbs

---

Figure 4: Conventional Confirmation of the Diagnoses of Type II Diabetes Mellitus

Fasting Sugar Level (no intake for at least 8 hrs):
- < 110: Normal
- >110 and < 126: Impaired Sugar Metabolism
- > 126: Patient has diabetes

An additional test is to administer sugar orally and then test your levels after 2 hours:
- <140: Normal
- >140 and <200: Impaired Sugar Metabolism
- >200: Patient has diabetes
- Random sugar level >200 along with symptoms of diabetes: Means patient has diabetes

TESTIMONIAL:

My name is Larry. I am a truck driver with diabetes. When I came to Dr. Ashworth's clinic to look into his program I was on the verge of losing my job due to my sugar levels being too high. Thanks to his program that involved changing my eating habits (eating times/portions/types of foods) and an exercise schedule, over a 6 month period I went from 308lbs to 250lb, JUST UNDER 60 POUNDS! This change gave me much more energy and of course a noticeable difference of lightness on my feet, not to even mention the changes it made in my diabetes status.

Dr. Ashworth worked with me every week; most of the time meeting me outside of normal working hours on Sundays (try to get most doctors to meet you on a Sunday!) because of my truck driving schedule. He tweaked my eating and exercise routines to fit an ever changing work schedule. I am still using those new habits he and his program helped me change and I'm still driving today. I would recommend this program to any person that wants to lose weight and improve their health and self esteem.

Larry

Figure 5: The major effects of Insulin that hinder weight management
- Makes you hungry
- Stimulates storage of fat
- Inhibits the breakdown of fat

The majorities of people who get Type II Diabetes are the ones with the "apple" shape and store their fat in their abdomen. In the past, we used to think fat was just a storage macro-nutrient that did very little. Now we now know that the abdominal fat releases a number of really nasty players. One of them is called Resistin. Resistin makes you "resistant" to the effects of insulin, requiring an increased amount of insulin to be produced by the pancreas to remove sugar from your blood and transport that sugar into your cells. Increased levels of insulin can also cause high blood pressure. Fat cells also release molecules that cause inflammation called IL-1, IL-6, and Tumor Necrosis Factor Alpha. These strange words basically mean this: you have constant inflammation in your body, suffer from constant fatigue, have stiff, sore joints, and get depressed a great deal of the time. People taking anti-depressants need to understand that their depression may drastically improve when they lose weight. I am certainly not saying that everyone who loses weight can discontinue their anti-depressants. To the contrary, I have found it necessary to write prescriptions for these medications during the weight management process and continue them after the patient has lost the weight. What I do believe is that the overweight or obese condition can make the feelings of depression worse.

Subcutaneous fat (the fat that you can pinch from the outside) is not the major player in insulin resistance. It is the fat under your abdominal muscles, the visceral adipose tissue as we call it. That is why "apple" shaped patients who have little fat that they can pinch are more susceptible to Type II diabetes. I have patients that need to lose the same amount of weight as an "apple" shaped person, but their weight is distributed on their hips, buttocks and legs. Most of the time these "pear" shaped people do not suffer from all of the metabolic problems that the "apple" shaped patients suffer from.

On the other hand the "pear" shaped women, or the ones with the lower body fat, have a much harder time getting the weight off. They do not have the disease processes, but they stay overweight longer. The "apple" shaped patients have an easier time getting the weight off once I have the insulin under control and are exercising. The major player of this scenario is an elevated insulin level that may be masking an underlying blood sugar problem. Remember it is not good that the sugar is under control if it is simply convincing the patient and their doctor that all is well. **To make THE DIAGNOSIS of diabetes early, measure insulin levels not sugar levels!** Once the diagnosis is made and treatment started, that is the time to keep track of sugar levels.

Figure 6: Diagnosis of Metabolic Syndrome (or Syndrome X)
- High fasting blood sugars
- High triglycerides, Low HDL (HDL is responsible for picking up the cholesterol and taking it back to the liver to be disposed of) that is why we as doctors like to see a high HDL
- High blood pressure
- Elevated waist to hip ratio/BMI of >29.9 in other words being Obese
- Small vessel coronary heart disease

The key is to not waste time and get the ball rolling towards losing the weight before things really get out of hand. Most patients do not like it when I tell them that they already have diabetes. Unfortunately it is true. They do have diabetes, and I want them to understand this because in many cases it will give them that little something extra, some of that "medical motivation" that may be needed to make it to their goal. When the normal range for sugar levels is 60-100 and someone comes in and their fasting sugar level is 95, they say they are not diabetic yet. Actually, a normal fasting blood sugar should be in the ball park of 70-80. If the person had steadily gained weight over a specified period of time, and the lab results over this same time frame showed an increasing fasting sugar level, it seems pretty obvious to me the trend is pointing to an insulin resistant state.

I tell them that if they really want a confirmation on that **diagnosis,** I could measure their insulin level and it would most likely be elevated. Insulin levels above 5 have historically indicated insulin resistance. That number actually makes sense when one considers the fact that the person has not had any food over the last 12 hours. Insulin is secreted when food enters the body; since food has not been eaten I would expect the insulin level to be almost non-existent. It is understandable then that when I saw the "Normal Ranges" for insulin that have started to become more prevalent were in the range of 0-25, I was shocked and irritated to say the least! Who benefits by changing lab levels that would certainly make it more likely that an increased number of individuals would not be diagnosed with insulin resistance until it was too late?

Because of this late diagnosis many of these people would end up causing more damage to their pancreas than needed. This in turn would all but guarantee future profits from this additional number of diabetics placed on medications.

I realize this sounds very "conspiracy theory" in nature, but I would rather believe my colleagues have been brain washed by the evil big pharma than believe they could be this ignorant to the obvious. I am not just being a blow hard either. I have treated these patients in the exact way I explain and have been able to help rid them of the extra pounds and the diabetic condition. HAVING AN ELEVATED DAY-LONG INSULIN LEVEL MAKES IT NEARLY IMPOSSIBLE TO GET WEIGHT OFF! Again, not being told why and how to make reducing weight easier reiterates the name of this book, "It's not your fault".

Diabetes, Insulin, and a word on Depression:

People who are overweight are often the first to tell me they are depressed. The person usually believes that it is most likely the result of them just not liking themselves. **The fact is (AND THIS IS AN IMPORTANT FACT) that one of the many harmful things that insulin resistance does is makes it difficult for the body to naturally produce serotonin from tryptophan!** Serotonin is one of the "feel good" chemicals in the brain that medicines like Prozac and Effexor try to increase our available supply of in the brain. For diabetics, staying away from high glycemic index carbohydrates is critical. There is a vicious cycle at work here. People who are overweight or obese usually understand the physical implications this confers upon them. They worry and stress about how to get the weight off and depression can easily set in. This is compounded by the reduction in serotonin that results from the increased concentration of insulin in the blood. This depression can become overwhelming and it needs to be addressed early on when treating this disease known as obesity. There is a chapter in the book completely dedicated to reversing this cycle. For now understand that there are many foods that are covered in this book that actually temporarily increase levels of these feel good hormones like serotonin and dopamine. Wait, ingesting substances that temporarily make a person feel good? Hmmm . . . this sounds strangely familiar. To be continued . . .

The Insulin Resistant "Funnel Effect":

Ok, back to sugar and insulin. As the sugar level increases, aside from telling us the pancreas is basically wearing out what harm does extra sugar do? When sugar (or glucose) is not handled properly because of insulin resistance, it eventually becomes attached to proteins in the blood. This is called glycosylation. One of the many end results is numb toes, an inability to heal sores on your lower extremities in general, and eventual amputation of these extremities. What is the process by which the decrease in blood flow occurs? Think of your blood vessels like tiny funnels. They start out with a larger opening as they leave the heart and get smaller and smaller as they branch out extending to the distant parts of the body. Sugar is supposed to be present in the blood. The problems begin when this sugar does not get removed from the blood. As a person stays insulin resistant, these extra sugars form little; let's just call them, "rocks". These "rocks" are proteins that become attached to sugar and at the very end of this funnel the rock cannot make it through the one cell layer thick opening that leads into the vein, which is the other funnel that leads back to the heart and lungs to pick up more oxygen. Yes, the passageway from an artery to the vein that leads back to the heart and lungs is only one cell layer thick. This is the start of cardiovascular disease or clogged arteries. The process occurs not only in the toes but everywhere in the body. That is why diabetes is known to be so damaging. This is the case even when your cholesterol levels look good.

Commercial labs have tried to corner the market in measuring very small cholesterol particles that they claim is the major cause of cardiovascular disease when the more traditional cholesterol levels are normal. I would argue that in overweight or obese people it is not these "low-density" cholesterol particles as much as these molecules I have discussed, these combinations of proteins and left over sugar that clog the arteries. These "rocks" just start to pile up in the arteries that carry oxygen and nutrients to the most distant parts of your body; your toes, the ends of blood vessels in your eyes (called retinopathy when in a diseased state), and the small filters in your kidneys (called nephropathy). As the funnel gets fuller, the amount of oxygen enriched blood and/or medicines; even medicines administered by IV to heal a wound can no longer reach those distant parts of your body and those parts of the body suffer. These nerves downstream of the blocked arteries start to scream out with pain, which is referred to as neuropathy in the legs (another big business in the pharmaceutical industry). This pain occurs because the nerves that are distal or downstream from the blockage are not getting the necessary oxygen and nutrients nerves require staying healthy. People can go blind and their kidneys can fail if this condition is left unchecked.

Part of the process of checking to see how long sugar has been floating around is to get a Hemoglobin A1c (HgB A1C) level. The present "normal range" for an HgB A1C level has been around for a long time and I have a serious problem using it to define, treat or diagnose diabetes. This is one of those labs that essentially tell the doctor the level of damage being inflicted on their patients' body. It is a very reactive lab. The only reasonable way to treat diabetes is to discover the elevated insulin levels and slowly rising sugar levels much earlier. This way we can begin the process of increasing the insulin sensitivity, clearing the blood of sugar, losing the necessary weight, and avoiding the diagnosis of diabetes all together.

There is good news and bad news. The bad news is that there is not an infinite life span on the pancreas. If it is left overworked too long it will never be able to fully recover and the patient may not be able to get off of their medications, primarily their injectable insulin. The good news is that diabetes does not have to be a life sentence. I have been able to take numerous patients completely off of their insulin. In most cases, the amount of insulin required to be injected decreases at incredible rates as their weight comes down, and they continue to exercise, eat appropriately, and drink their water. This entire process is way out of the scope of a simple commercial weight loss center. We need more doctors like me who understand how to manage these disease processes. The good news is that if the disorder has not been overlooked too long there is a high likelihood that each person will be able to completely come off all of their medications and recover from diabetes.

A diabetic patient example:

I was recently told about a person who is a good friend of a present patient. He is one of those men who go to see their doctor only when they feel sick. This person was obese, but did not have any overt medical problems aside from some bluish discoloration in their lower legs. Their legs also tended to be progressing to a less than stellar sensitivity to the touch. Not to mention their toes seemed to be tingling and at times seemed to go completely numb. He had gone to his primary care doctor 5 years prior and at that time was overweight. He had basic lab panels ran and all seemed well, according to his doctor at the time. The doctor did mention that his cholesterol was high and that his FASTING BLOOD SUGAR was very near <u>the upper limit of normal</u>. His insulin level was never measured. Five years later the friend of this overweight diabetic is talking to me in my clinic and telling me his story. He now has extremely poor circulation in both lower extremities, decreased sensation and his blood sugars are now elevated! Well I hate to write this again, but if he had simply had his insulin level measured earlier, the diagnosis of diabetes could have been made, the proper medications prescribed and the damage to the pancreas, and lower extremity blood flow circumvented. But hey the doctor did all he was required to do by way of the "Standard of Care" so why the complaining? A paradigm shift is needed; the "Standard of Care" needs a higher standard.

How to treat Diabetes:

As the patient gets their insulin levels down, they will be able to lose weight faster! This is a great double whammy for most people. They are glad that they have to stick themselves less <u>and</u> they are finally reducing weight. Weight management is much easier once the insulin is out of the way or at least consistently reduced. Oral medications vary in my ability to remove them early. I like to get patients off of the medications that force the pancreas to make more insulin. These medications are referred to as glucosurias: Glyburide or Glucotrol. As I said, these are usually first line therapy when a patient fails to lose weight with exercise, eating less, and following a basic, copied, and stored in your doctors top drawer 1200 calories diabetic diet. Yes you read that correctly. Even though the root problem for the constant weight gain is the elevated insulin, first line therapy for many doctors is to start a medication that squeezes out more insulin to be dumped into the blood stream.

These types of medications just make weight management harder and increase the chance that your sugars may drop too low on a low carbohydrate, lower calorie weight management program. On the other hand, the medications that help make you more sensitive to insulin, like metformin, are the best to continue using or begin to use. Medications like metformin help the process and need to be taken as long as you are trying to lose weight as long as they are not contraindicated which needs to be confirmed by your doctor. My goal is to make your pancreas more efficient and have to work less, so it lasts longer. We want the day-long insulin levels to be lower. This will help us keep the weight coming off consistently and metformin will accomplish this.

There is a specific protocol to decrease insulin as a person is reducing weight and decreasing their calories. It is up to your doctor to understand this process. Every doctor's goal should be to try and help their patient lose the weight, cure their diabetes, and help them decrease their intake of medications as a whole. Diabetes is a killer, and it needs to be the focus early on. If you have a lot of abdominal fat get your fasting insulin levels measured early, as well as your fasting sugar levels to watch for trends. Encourage your doctor to help you aggressively lose weight or refer you to someone that will. It will never be as simple as giving you an appetite suppressant (which I do not have a problem using), a 1200 calorie diabetic diet, and telling you to go lose weight.

I have cured many patients of this disease. Do not let anyone tell you it is a life sentence until you have been thoroughly examined by a weight management medicine doctor. It is a heredity problem in many cases. If your parents were overweight and ended up with diabetes and you are overweight, then you are in a higher risk category for the diabetic condition. If you have been seen by a doctor who has ignored the warning signs I have written about and you already have diabetes, you need help. It is <u>not your fault</u> that the weight will not come off. You will just need an aggressive approach by a doctor dedicated to helping their patients get the weight off. It takes time to deal with both weight management and the diseases it causes. In these situations I would advise the physicians in your area that have obese patients, and do not practice aggressive weight management medicine to find a doctor that specializes in this and refer to that doctor.

TESTIMONIAL:

I would like to take the time to thank Dr. Lance Ashworth and his staff at Ashworth Medical Solutions for their continued support and guidance during my weight management. I had just been diagnosed with Type II Diabetes Mellitus and was also experiencing a lot of the fatigue, depression, and lack of menstruation that go with hormone disorders. Type 2 Diabetes is not an easy thing to accept at first and also experiencing the emotional swings that go with peri-menopause did not help.

With the aid of Dr. Ashworth's weight management plan, his bio-identical hormone replacement therapy regimen, and proper medications I was able to lose 70 pounds! I'm not saying there weren't any struggles or trials, but going to see him regularly and listening to his encouraging words helped me get closer to my goal of 100 pounds of weight management.

As a non-food reward, I asked Dr. Ashworth if he would perform Liposculpting on me. The results are phenomenal, and were able to be noticed just days after the swelling went down, and it was painless! I thank you and all of your patience with me as I struggled through losing weight with diabetes and discovering all of the hormone imbalances I had that you corrected. Today I have a new and happier life especially after having the Liposculpting he performs as a cosmetic surgeon! In time, I am sure I will be able to get off all of my medications once I also lose the fat that is under my abdominal muscles.

I look forward to continuing my weight management journey. I want to lose another 30-40 pounds which doesn't seem like such a far off goal having so many parts of my life back in MY control. I would probably be on insulin right now if it wasn't for your weight management program. Thank you again and I will see you soon.

Susan

All of my insulin dependent diabetics get my personal cell phone number in the beginning of the weight management process. As they are decreasing their insulin intake, I have them call me with their daily sugar readings two to three times per day. They do not get an answering service—they get me. I help them with the process of safely lowering their dosages of insulin to avoid dangerous drops in sugar. This is the sort of commitment you need from your doctor when you are reducing weight and diabetes is being dealt with.

The first time I actually saw the words "Diabetes Resolved" was when I wrote these words in a patient's chart. I actually wondered if I was allowed to write it! During my medical training, I usually saw "increase this diabetic medication" or "diabetes under control, or needs to be under tighter control". I always suspected there was a better way. It may not be the easiest way, but understanding how insulin can make things difficult and focusing on this hormone gives patients hope that there is a solid place to start. A problem that once we get handled will not only help with weight management, but the cycle will finally start to be broken. When you lose weight, the insulin level drops and you get less hungry, eat less and lose more weight. Insulin will then drop some more, you have to take less medicine, and the process keeps going in this positive direction. This also sounds like a cycle, but a cycle most diabetics would love to be in.

After adjustment of the medications, the next step is to eat the correct type of foods during the process of weight management. This is accomplished by choosing low glycemic index (GI) foods, foods that are digested more slowly. Having food to eat during the weight management process is a weight management program that is going in the right direction. We will always need to eat, and learning from the very start to eat the right foods in the right amounts is important. A solid 10-15% of our resting metabolic rate is solid food digestion. It is important early on to learn to handle portion and stimulus control.

Stimulus control was first studied at Harvard. They found that when dealing with food limiting the variety, amount, color, smell and whatever else can be controlled will help the person eat less. So the goal is to avoid being stimulated by a large variety of foods during the weight management "Active Weight Reduction Phase". I like to have solid food in my programs, as opposed to full liquid diets, because of the routine of controlling what and how much we eat. I do occasionally use what is referred to as a "Protein Sparing Modified Fast" (PSMF). This type of medically supervised program uses five 160 calorie shakes that have a full complement of vital nutrients and vitamins. I reserve this sort of program for patients that have a lot of weight to lose and would like a jump start in the beginning. It is limited to 60 days and then I add solid food back in and continue the program. I will also use a PSMF with those people that want to lose 40 pounds or less and have no major health concerns. I call this program the "60/40 Modified Medical Fast", where the person can lose 40 pounds in 60 days. In diabetics I always use solid food in the program because it makes it easier to predict and control insulin and sugar.

All of my programs end with a transition phase. This is a 4-6 week transition where the medical shakes are removed from the program and solid food replaces that caloric equivalent. I do not want the program a person uses to drop weight to be so different from what they will be on the rest of their life. So since they will be eating the rest of their life, I want them eating some solids either throughout the entire program or towards the end on the weight management programs that I provide. It is vital that your doctor understands the art of compromise. Not every patient is the same and some patients tell me they are having an extremely hard time controlling their portion sizes of food and need a break from food altogether. This is a time when I may start them on a PSMF that contains no solids for 30-60 days if they meet the requirements.

The strength behind using low glycemic index foods is that they travel through the intestinal tract slowly, being digested slowly, hence entering the bloodstream in the same way. With all of the damage insulin can do at high levels, we need to do everything possible to keep the day-long insulin levels as close to normal as possible. This is why I have included a list of foods that are low LGI choices. Use these foods often while building your food program based on the information you will learn in this book. However, our goal will be to control insulin in every way possible from what you put in your mouth, to how much lean muscle you build along the way. Both play major roles in helping control this vital hormone.

You need to know the basics. IMPORTANT POINT: You need to understand enough to ask the correct questions that prompt actions by your doctor that will hopefully result in a sincere interest in incorporating weight management medicine into your treatment and their practice.

> **Figure 7: What should be used for insulin sensitivity to include both Rx and OTC?**
> - Metformin- <u>A prescription medication</u> taken at 500 mg once or twice per day, which increases insulin sensitivity in the skeletal muscles and decreases sugar production by the liver.
> - Alpha Lipoic Acid at 50 mg/day OTC
> - Conjugated Linoleic Acid at 500 mg/day OTC
> - Chromium at 400-800 mg/day OTC
> - Methionine at 500 mg/day OTC
> - Inositol at 500 mg/day OTC
> - Choline at 250 mg/day OTC

Some conservative over-the-counter insulin sensitizers as listed in the figure above are alpha lipoic acid at 50 mg/day, conjugated linoleic acid at 500 mg/day, and chromium at 400-800 mg/day. Methionine 500 mg/day, Inositol 500 mg/day, and choline 250 mg/day are three others that can have an impact on your ability to lose weight. These last three, along with the injectable form of HSL-Accelerator™ (described in Appendix: E) are combined in my practice and given as an intra-muscular injection. Not only do they increase insulin sensitivity, but they give the patient the energy they need to get out and exercise. Methionine and inositol are great insulin sensitizers. Choline is pulled out of the blood when muscles are contracting to be used in the creation of acetylcholine, which enables them to continue to contract. As this choline is pulled out of the blood, more acetylcholine is able to be made and the muscles continue to contract, hence burning fat. Weight management needs to be approached from every angle. What you deserve is for every physician to attack this disease with the same fervor.

What patients need to understand is that once they have full blown diabetes requiring insulin, it is not the end of the road for them. It is true that weight management is tougher until the amount of injected insulin is reduced. When a person starts weight management the first reduction in insulin is usually a cut in half! My job is to get as much of that insulin out of the way as quickly as possible so weight reduction is as quick as possible. Patients are amazed by the reduction in their daily insulin requirements when they are consistently eating low glycemic index foods (the good carbohydrates), drinking water, exercising regularly, and drinking their medical shakes!

The obvious question at this point is how to control the blood sugars? ***Let us be clear on one point***: when the cuts are made in the insulin intake, I want the sugar readings to be higher. **That is OK!** We are not talking about off the chart sugar levels. But because the calorie counts are lower than what the body is accustomed to experience has taught that keeping the sugars in the range of 150-200 during the Active Weight Reduction Phase is the safest. I am not talking over the long term, just during this initial phase. Believe me when I say that these sugar readings will not be elevated long. After the body becomes more insulin sensitive and we reduce the insulin injected, and at weight reduction of 3-5 pounds per week the sugars begin to normalize in 90-120 days. The patients are surprised that I am fine with readings that come in over 200. I would much rather you wake up in the morning after eating a day's worth of low sugar items, vegetables, water, and drinking shakes at a total calorie count that at times can be as low as 1000. This is much more desirable than keeping a person on the same dose of insulin and have sugars drop below 40 sending the person into a diabetic coma that night. If they will just concentrate on being a compliant patient and do what I tell them to do, the weight management can be tremendous. While the rest of the world is talking about the alarming rate in the increase of diabetes, I concentrate on how many patients I can place in the "diabetes resolved" category.

I am not writing this book so you the reader can determine how much food to eat, and attempt to reduce medications or your insulin dosage on your own. Remember, there is not a book written that could possibly apply to everyone. Even though I firmly stand behind the protocols outlined in this book, the type and amount of insulin you should be taking and reducing will vary from person to person. This book is being published so you can convince your doctor that there is a better, more thorough way to treat patients that are overweight and suffering with these conditions. Sure, there are a few things I have included in the book that you as the reader can implement on your own. But the change I am looking for is the one where doctors take some time out of their week and dedicate it to treating their overweight/obese population of patients. This is a huge step for most doctors, but one that absolutely has to be made. The general practice and internal medicine doctors are at the front lines. It is time for them to take up arms and defeat this enemy we call obesity. One thing I need to say though is that if you do convince your doctor to take up the fight, you need to be a compliant patient and do what he/she needs you to do to get the job done.

TESTIMONIAL:

My life has been spent trying to help and please others. Consequently, my excuse for my lack of exercise and discipline was also my codependency. At Christmas-time, my family began to really talk to me about my long term health. With my first grandchild on the way, I became excited about the days of fun and engagement in activity with this little one, which I already loved dearly. My wife said, "Larry if you don't do something about your health, you won't be around to enjoy this little one. I want you to grow old with me, and the kids are worried about you." Those words hit me like an anvil being dropped on my heart, I knew they were true. At the time, my blood pressure had soared to 158/110; I was on daily medication for hypertension. My blood sugar levels were at high normal. My cholesterol was way out of whack. Constant back, neck and shoulder pain were really minimizing my quality of life. Minor activity would cause shortness of breath and heavy perspiration. I also struggled to sleep because of sleep apnea for which I was being treated. It had been a long time since I had enjoyed much of the benefits of physical activity; softball is no fun at 262 pounds.

None of these consequences for my choices even begins to explain how I felt about myself inside. On the inside I despised myself. From a well conditioned athlete through college to where I had allowed myself to decline was personally appalling. Recently moving to Florida, I decided to look on the internet for some help. I believe through God's blessing I ran across the Ashworth Medical website and decided to stop by and ask questions. Stevie was my first contact, and before leaving I scheduled an appointment to see Dr. Ashworth. When I came for my first visit and interview, I was greeted by some of the most positive and encouraging office staff I could imagine. Now they all seem like personal buddies and allies through the journey. They were always full of encouragement and compliments, no matter how little my success at times. Life sometimes gets in the way of doing things perfectly. I never left one time feeling discouraged though. The Staff was merely a reflection of Dr. Ashworth. He was a guy I could relate to. He was a "Let's get it done" kind of a guy. The personal confidence backed up by his obvious success in health really gave me a sense of hope. Dr Ashworth never talked about only treating symptoms, but discussed my cure! I was going to be healthy again; he had convinced me it could be done. All the support and accountability I so desperately needed I found in the weekly check-ups and group meetings loaded with information.

After I decided to be a part of his program, he asked me what would keep me going. Early I said, "Because I am determined, and when I have a goal, I won't waste it." Later on I realized my real motivation, I really like feeling and looking great. I wouldn't trade the life I have now for anything. Today I have lost over 75 pounds and am healthier than I have been in years. The hypertension is gone, the blood sugar is normal, and I can walk briskly for an hour and not be winded. My chronic back, neck and shoulder pain is gone. My confidence and self-worth are what they ought to be. Begin a journey that will end in the best days of your life!

Larry

Testimonials such as this one are fantastic to read and I will never tire of helping people reach their goals. But the goal for me is to change the thought and treatment patterns of physicians around the globe. This will be realized when you can walk into any clinic and find a physician that has learned how to medically treat weight issues and joined the fight against obesity, the number one preventable disease. A fight I have stood alone in for too many years.

> *POW:* *IF YOU HAVE BEEN OVERWEIGHT FOR AWHILE, YOU GAINED THAT WEIGHT IN YOUR MIDSECTION, AND YOUR BLOOD SUGARS HAVE STEADILY RISEN; IT IS IMPERATIVE YOU TELL YOUR DOCTOR TO START MEASURING YOUR INSULIN LEVELS INSTEAD!*

CHAPTER 5

Our Sex Hormones: Deficiencies
and how to correct them

The Women's Health Initiative Experimental Trial:

The Women's Health Initiative Trial, which was stopped in June of 2002, looked at conventional hormone replacement therapy (HRT) which included a combination of Premarin and Provera. Thousands of women had been followed in this study for years in an attempt to measure the effects that these two hormones had on the women. Premarin is a synthetic estrogen made from pregnant horse mare urine, actually 40% of Premarin is estrogen derived from pregnant horse mare urine, which being from a horse is very difficult for the human body to recognize or metabolize. I don't have a problem per say with horses; I just do not want their chemically altered urine in my wife or daughters in the future.

Provera, or medroxyprogesterone acetate, is a synthetic progestin. Many physicians refer to Provera as progesterone. <u>Provera is not the same as progesterone.</u> Synthetic progestin, such as those found in Provera and other progestins that were looked at in the WHI study, showed an increase in the risk of breast cancer; whereas, natural progesterone made by the body is <u>actually</u> breast cancer protective. A great example of this would be to look at a time when women were at their highest biological levels of progesterone, in their mid twenties. If there was going to be any time that progesterone would cause cancer it would most likely be when the levels were at their highest. Yet very few women are fighting breast cancer in this age range. Not a very strong argument for progesterone being the causative effect of breast cancer. Yes, progesterone is breast cancer protective. Take a second to read those last few sentences again.

Synthetic progestin's also increase the risk of heart disease. Provera has been shown to be a coronary vasoconstrictor, which means that it narrows the blood vessels that supply blood and oxygen to the heart muscle. Natural or bio-identical progesterone, on the other hand, acts as a coronary vasodilator opening up the blood vessels. Synthetic progestin's are not protective against osteoporosis or bone loss like natural progesterone. Synthetic progestin's can cause fluid retention also. On the other hand, progesterone is a natural diuretic (it helps the body get rid of excess water!).

Synthetic progestin's can cause weight gain. Natural or what we refer to as bio-Identical progesterone helps burn fat for energy and balances insulin and cortisol, which also aids with weight control. No wonder it was so much easier to lose weight when you were younger! The synthetic progestin's found in the birth control pill and conventional HRT can cause depression. Progesterone is a natural antidepressant and calming hormone. Just think of the name of the hormone pro-gesterone: literally pro-gestation, keep the baby, stay calm and keep the uterus calm.

The trial (WHI) was actually stopped early because of the findings. The researchers found a 41 % increase in strokes, a 29% increase in heart attacks, a 26% increase in the incidence of breast cancer, and twice the rate of pulmonary embolism (blood clots to the lungs) and blood clots in the legs. It was not a surprise that oral conventional HRT increased the risk of breast cancer, strokes, and blood clots because there was already evidence in the medical literature (but hey they were FDA approved right). The researchers also felt that the combination of Premarin and Provera contributed to the development of Alzheimer's disease. The study showed a decrease in the incidence of colon cancer and hip fractures. The authors felt that the synthetic progestin called Provera was the main culprit in the complications. Another arm of the trial looked at

Premarin (synthetic estrogen) alone. The only statistically significant complication was a slight (.12%) increase in the risk of strokes. Personally I think women would have rather put up with the hot flashes and night sweats that these medications prevented, since the medicines really did nothing else aside from causing an early death, but that is just me.

Bio-Identical Hormones:

In the beginning of my career the defining moment, the most significant breakthrough for me as a weight management physician came when I began studying bio-identical hormones. A hormone is a chemical messenger that may act on its own or it may be responsible for releasing other hormones. These bio-identical hormones literally leveled the playing field between women and men 35 years old and up when compared to those of the same gender 34 and below in ages. Women are tired of being told they're just going to have to expect that all of those post-menopausal symptoms are a part of growing older. Or that gaining weight and getting wrinkles are just part of the process of adding on those years. Men are equally as tired hearing that part of growing older includes a decrease in their sex drive as well as their sexual performance. That their lack of energy, and diminishing amount of lean muscle, increasing aches and pains, as well as slow recovery from exercise are inevitable and unavoidable.

I will agree that it is harder to lose weight when one grows older, but aside from other diagnoses you will also read about, this difficulty is for the most part caused by a decrease in hormone production by either the ovaries or testicles and there is a solution! The solution is bio-identical replacement of those hormones. We age and gain weight more easily because our hormones are slowly depleting and if we are going to fight back then we need to consider the option of bio-identical HRT. These hormones are not new; it has just been very difficult to compete with the deep advertising budgets of large pharmaceutical companies that advertise their patented synthetic hormones. It's a good thing bio-identical hormones are available because what options would men and women have? Especially when most of the obstetricians and gynecologists in this country are still to this day completely against any sort of bio-identical alternative to the synthetic hormone replacement they have handed out like candy for decades. The same synthetic therapy that the Women's' Health Initiative (WHI) showed us are dangerous. The only major difference now is that the gynecologists will take you off of them after 5 years. Well, sooner if you get cancer or blood clots before that 5 year mark. Even if those hot flashes and night sweats return, you will still be advised not to take anything. Why will they still prescribe them, or offer nothing? Because these synthetic drugs are FDA approved of course, and that must make them safer than anything else not yet approved . . . . right? Wrong.

Whether a compound is "natural" or "synthetic" is not the issue. The molecular shape and structure must be identical to what is made in the human body to not only fit into the appropriate receptor, but also render the same effect in the body as the hormone which the body naturally produced. In today's common usage, "synthetic" has come to mean "artificial," but this is not always correct. Synthetic simply means "produced by a method outside of the body." So "natural" or bio-identical hormones are made in the laboratory, and the process is called "synthesizing." The source of these hormones are yam and wild soy beans. The carbons and hydrogen's in these two plants are able to be "synthesized" to not only fit into the correct receptors in the human body, but start the resulting chemical reactions in the cells they attach to that is helpful and healthy instead of harmful. And they help with a whole lot more than just reducing hot flashes and night sweats.

A dangerous aspect of the synthesizing process in the case of estrogen, or more commonly known as Premarin is that it is from the urine of a pregnant mare. This medication turns out to be a mixture of estrogens found in a "natural" state, *albeit that of a different species*. The problem was that many of these estrogens are not found "naturally" in the human body. So let us just call a horse a horse . . . no let's not. This mixture of estrogens has been found to have many dire consequences for women who take it. They were led to believe that they were taking 17-beta estradiol even though all of those FDA approved long term studies never confirmed this very important fact. My belief is that if there was money to be made in the use of bio-identical hormones and a couple of pharmaceutical companies came out with their own versions it would not be long before pharmaceutical representatives would have magically changed their sales pitch.

It is surprising how many health care providers do not comprehend the vast difference between synthetic chemical substitutes and the body's natural hormones, at least in terms of how they refer to them by name when talking to the patient they are about to prescribe them for. I know they know the difference they just don't seem to emphasize it when prescribing it. I would say that a thorough explanation is in order since progestin actually has a lot of the opposite effects the patient is looking for. In the end it's your job to ask! Doctors may tell you that progesterone made from Yams and Soy are also synthetic, because they are broken down and made just like we have had to "make" progestin. You simply agree, because it is true. It's just that the way they put their carbons and hydrogen's back together to make progestin and Premarin kills us instead of helps us! So why did manufacturing companies make them this way? Because it was a cheaper method to produce these medicines and they were able to be patented. So simply say you'd rather go with the "not going to make me the breast cancer or stroke victim version" of synthetic!

The serious conditions caused by obesity, like stroke among many others, are unacceptable in my view. Many physicians will spout off the absence of studies that show the effectiveness of BHRT. The most ridiculous aspect of this "absence of a long term study" reasoning, especially among gynecologist's, in the majority of cases is that these doctors have not sought them out and read them. Just because they have not been spoon fed the study by a pharmaceutical representative does not mean the studies are non-existent!

TESTIMONIAL:

I have been a patient of Dr. Ashworth's since July of 2007 for weight management. Being 53 years old, exercising regularly, and having tried numerous diets, I was at 249 pounds and unable to lose any weight—and I continued to see the additional weight gain year after year. I had a complete abdominal hysterectomy in 2000 and was on hormone medication. I had also been diagnosed with hypothyroidism several years ago by my family physician and was taking Synthroid for that condition.

The first thing Dr. Ashworth did was look at some basic labs and change my thyroid medication to Armour Thyroid, in addition to starting his program of shakes three times a day, combined with low glycemic index foods. After 4 months, I had lost 30 pounds! This wasn't quite as fast as he would have liked so he performed a complete hormone lab evaluation; Dr. Ashworth discovered that my hormone levels were virtually non-existent. He then started me on his Bio-Identical Hormone Replacement Therapy (BHRT) program, to increase these necessary hormone levels. The reason why he waited was because I was a bit afraid of going in that direction with all of the bad press about hormone therapy. Since starting BHRT, I no longer have to take hormones in a pill format (basically those synthetic hormones). It has helped me sleep better and I am able to exercise for longer periods of time. And I don't have to worry about hot flashes, either.

I've now lost just over 50 pounds—and I want to continue to lose more. It is so exciting to not only lose the weight—finally— but be able to keep it off. What is great about Dr. Ashworth is that he tailors his program to the individual. If something is not working, or if the weight management has stagnated, he goes the extra mile to find the cause and correct it.

Sincerely, DH, Ormond Beach, Fl

Granted these Bio-Identical Hormones are not the fountain of youth, Ok they very well may be, but even if they are not they sure make the quality of life better as we live longer. We do not have to live with becoming obese, contracting diabetes or being held captive in our homes because of all of the aches and pains we are wracked with as our naturally produced hormones decline. As we grow older the hormone deficiencies just creep up on us. We do not just wake up one morning and say, "Wow I feel like crap. My hormones must be depleted." It is more of an insidious and slow depletion that is difficult to notice. We just get used to feeling as we do and assume it is normal. Many physicians just tell their patients that it is a part of getting older and there is very little to do about it. At least the doctor gets the general idea of the diagnosis, we are getting older. They are just missing the other 99% of what is going on with their patient and what can be done hormonally to improve their patient's health. They not only need to understand the importance of these hormones, but understand the concept of dosing these hormones. For years the standard of care was that if a woman was experiencing hot flushes, night sweats, etc. they were put on one of two doses of usually Premarin. There was no blood test to determine what dose of this estrogen to administer based on the persons present levels. No effort was made to figure out if their weight would affect the effectiveness of the dose. It was not an issue to consider the implications of un-opposed estrogen therapy. This simply means giving a woman estrogen without any effort to also give progesterone providing balance. The bottom line was that if a woman had undergone a hysterectomy and their uterus was absent why would they need progesterone? I suppose they just assumed all progesterone was good for was helping to sustain the lining of the uterus during pregnancy. Did it occur to anyone that since progesterone helped calm the uterus and sustain the pregnancy, might it not also be involved in a calming effect on the body when the woman is not pregnant? Could it possibly be involved in helping a woman sleep, avoid depression; be involved in weight gain in some way. These are just a couple of questions that can be asked of your doctor when and if you are considering hormone replacement therapy.

As you consider this know that I would go as far as to say that the hormones released by the ovaries, testacles, and <u>adrenals </u>without a doubt are the most important in terms of weight management and weight maintenance. People will tell me they are on a plan that allows them to lose weight slow so they do not gain the weight back. I could care less how slow someone loses their weight if the health problems, at the very least the ones' presented in this book are not addressed. This is because this slow weight reduction will mean very little and the weight will return no matter how slow they lose it, if medical problems are not addressed that contributed to the weight gain in the first place.

Actually let us use a common example of fast weight reduction that everyone seems to be fine with. How about the people who go get the Gastric-By Pass operation? No one seems to be overly concerned with the speed at which they lose weight, which is also on average 3-5 pounds per week. Any given month I will usually be treating a patient that has had this very operation and yes, they gained all, if not a significant portion of their weight back. There are a couple of reasons for this. Neither one of the reasons have anything to do with the speed that the weight was lost. The first and most important reason they gain weight back is if they did not have the medical or psychological problem leading to their weight gain diagnosed and properly treated. The second is that these people who undergo this operation usually are not prepared to follow the virtual laundry list of vitamins, minerals, nutrients, and the exceedingly small amounts of food they are required to eat numerous times per day to just stay healthy. In comparison to the hardest weight management program they could imagine, undergoing this operation and then staying at the weight or even attaining the weight they wish to get down to is much more difficult than most could have ever suspected.

Hormones in balance are the key to overall health. I realize that even considering hormone therapy is scary these days, but read on and you will be surprised. Dealing with the more commonly known disorders like hypothyroidism and diabetes is a great place to start, but in many cases may just be scratching the surface. This subject of HRT is a sensitive one to say the least. The Women's Health Initiative had everyone thinking that any and every hormone must be bad for us. The truth of the matter is that bio-identical hormones are completely different from the ones used in that study. In my clinic as the years went by, it became evident to me that women in menopause or ones who had a hysterectomy where the ovaries were also taken lost weight slower than other patients. These same women recovered from exercise slower or had a tougher time exercising. In general, they just seemed to deal with fat in a different way. One comment that seemed to be common among all of them was, "It never used to be this hard to lose weight when I was younger." So unless I was going to attempt to build a time machine, I knew their hormones probably held some answers.

As I began studying the positive benefits of these hormones, I knew that bio-identical hormone replacement did answer the many problems these patients were having with fatigue, weight management, decreasing libido, loss of lean muscle, and the myriad of other symptoms that go with declining hormone levels. My studies began to come together when I looked at the Adrenal Glands. We all have two adrenal glands, one on top of each kidney. Having two of the same type of gland led me to believe they must hold a very important piece of this hormone puzzle I was trying to understand. The next clue was the fact that the second hormone made from the adrenals was progesterone! These glands also produce estrogens, testosterone, as well as a host of others vital to our body. These glands held many of the answers I had been asking for a long time. The adrenals are what we come to depend on as we live past the child bearing years when these hormones are at their highest levels. So as we live longer we come to depend more on the adrenal hormones, but in much lower levels than what we required as younger men and women who were trying to conceive and raise children. The take home point or better yet, the take home question for me was why did the adrenals continue to make these hormones at all? The answer is that we absolutely continue to require these hormones but in much smaller amounts. The problem is that the adrenal glands are becoming fatigued in large percentages of people. This is because as we battle with all of the daily stressors in our lives the adrenals have to work overtime. They are in use not only in times of high life stressors, but are in high gear during times of sickness. Especially when dealing with long term illnesses. It seems as though stress has become an accepted part of all of our lives. Unfortunately this inevitably leads to what we call Adrenal Fatigue. The next section will deal exclusively in how to diagnose and treat Adrenal fatigue

As I began to realize the positive benefits of having at least an adrenal gland level of these hormones, I knew that bio-identical hormone replacement answered many of the problems these patients were experiencing. As with most of the disorders I investigate as a possibility of being the reason why weight gain is occurring, it starts with a blood test. Every person needs to have their hormones in balance, and it is a very important part in discovering why they are overweight. If a doctor is going to start helping people lose weight, the doctor better start studying bio-identical hormone replacement therapy (BHRT).

TESTIMONIAL:

When I first came to Dr. Ashworth I was very overweight and very depressed because no matter what I did, I could not lose weight. I was 56 years old at the time, and he was really my last resort. I had tried every crazy diet there was to no avail. I really prepared [myself] for the usual routine of some assistant checking your pulse and weighing you and then giving you a diet or some pills and sending you on your way. Boy was I surprised.

Dr. Ashworth spent our time together inquiring about my life, feelings, moods, and habits. Most importantly, he told me that it wasn't my entire fault that I couldn't lose weight or that I was feeling bad, not sleeping, etc. He told me about bio-identical hormone therapy. Now, I had been on hormones some years before when menopause started but went off of them because of all the scares. I wasn't totally sure I should go back on them, but I really came to trust Dr. Ashworth completely.

After getting complete blood work done and baseline readings, he started me on a regimen of estradiol, progesterone, and testosterone—all applied in a cream form. Eventually I started to use the pellet form of the estradiol and testosterone and just used the progesterone cream daily. This is what changed my life. I sleep at night soundly. My exercising actually shows results. I have lost inches where I never could lose them before. I actually lost weight while I was following a really healthy diet. My cholesterol count went down and my blood pressure decreased. My husband will tell you that the best thing that happened was that I got my sex drive back, so he is really grateful to Dr. Ashworth. My primary care physician and gynecologist were pleased with my weight management and improved overall medical status. When they asked me what I was doing I told them bio-identical HRT. Neither of them knew what I was talking about. Pretty sad!

R.S. Ormond Beach, Fl

How to treat sex hormone deficiencies with bio-identical hormones:

The Estrogens:

There are three major estrogens which are found in balance in a healthy female. These are **estrone (E1)**, **estradiol (E2)**, and **estriol (E3)**. An important point to remember is that estrogen when taken orally in a pill form can cause an increase in inflammation, and the dose you are prescribed is unreliable because it has to be metabolized by the liver; known as the "First Pass Effect" and each person metabolizes oral medicines at differing levels depending on physiology and medications they may take. I prefer the transdermal cream route or the use of a pellet form that is implanted in a fatty layer of the rear hip area.

Estradiol or **E2** is a strong estrogen and is the form of estrogen that is used in bio-identical HRT. High, unopposed, or out of balance levels may increase the risk of breast, uterine, and prostate cancer (in men). This is why it is vital that women *have progesterone as well as estrogen* when getting supplemented with bio-identical hormones. This is the case whether the woman has a uterus or not. Yes, whether the woman has a uterus or not. Certain amounts of estradiol are extremely important for the health of both women and men. It is vital for the health of the heart, brain, bones, joints, immune system, and much more.

Progesterone:

Progesterone, not the drug company's version called progestin or medroxyprogesteroneacetate, balances the other hormones in the body including the estrogens <u>and</u> insulin (the enemy to weight management!). It is critical to maintain hormonal balance which protects the breast, uterus, and in men the prostate gland. Having naturally low levels of progesterone have been associated with an increased risk of breast cancer. Progesterone also protects the brain, including injury from trauma and strokes. Progesterone promotes new bone formation by stimulating osteoblasts (cells in bone that promote bone growth when stimulated) and opens up the blood vessels around the heart. Progesterone also has a role in restoring libido along with testosterone. Here we see it again, an example of how all of our hormones work in concert when balanced.

After being in practice for a few years I received a phone call from one of the more prominent gynecologists in the area. She called at the behest of her patient who wanted her gynecologist's blessing for me to use the bio-identical hormones in her treatment. This was in part because the patient did not want to take any more of the premarin (or pregnant horse mare urine). The doctor said she did not have any problem with me using the hormones, because she wanted the woman to have a hysterectomy. I did not have any problems with a hysterectomy because it cuts down; in general, on the number of cancers a woman is at risk for, namely uterine, cervical, and ovarian. The only problem that was sure to arise once the uterus and cervix was removed would be the question as to why I wanted to continue or start progesterone on the post-hysterectomy female. This particular doctor, like so many other gynecologists, was sure to question the use of progesterone once the uterus is removed? Sure enough, once we got on the topic of a hysterectomy this doctor voiced the same objection as the others with the use of progesterone once the uterus was gone.

I could not resist it. All I had to do was tell my colleague to go look up the research. But, instead I hopped up on my soap box and began the diatribe on the benefits of progesterone whether or not she had a uterus. Five minutes later there was silence. Then she rattled off a few unsubstantiated risks. I then explained the importance of keeping the hormones in balance. I explained that progesterone actually increased the blood flow to the heart and was breast cancer protective. I said this is not hard to understand when the breast cancer and heart problems begin after the progesterone is gone. How many twenty one year olds have you seen with breast cancer? There are also the benefits of anti-anxiety and being able to actually sleep well at night. Silence reigned once again. Like she had fallen asleep; but I knew that was impossible because this doctor was also post-menopausal and didn't sleep any better than her patient. She then said "we will know more when additional studies come out." That's fine. These doctors need to understand though that the studies will not magically appear on their desks. They will need to seek out the studies and read them. Until then we can agree to disagree. Controversy is ok when it benefits the patient! The patient was smart enough to have the full complement of hormones, and decided she will continue with them whether she has a hysterectomy or not.

Testosterone:

Testosterone has a huge impact on a person's ability to drop weight and then maintain it. I come at weight management medicine from this angle primarily because I am a weight management doctor, but the number of mechanisms this hormone drives in men and women are too numerous to ignore. Because 30-40% of our lean body mass is muscle, and muscle can contribute up to 40% of a person's metabolism this is just one of the many reasons this hormone plays such a large part in weight management. With exercise playing such a major role in weight maintenance, and our muscles being the major player in participating in exercise, testosterones importance should not be a surprise. This hormone increases energy and the ability to build and maintain this lean muscle while shortening recovery time from exercise. All of these affect your metabolism and the ability to lose and then more importantly maintain the weight lost.

There are many other benefits of testosterone for both men and women. When in low levels, testosterone affects many aspects of our mental health, including libido. People do not normally associate testosterone with their mental activity, but their memory and ability to concentrate will diminish as the levels of testosterone diminish. Along with the total testosterone, the level of free testosterone is just as important to measure, especially when looking at protection from developing Alzheimer's and Parkinson's disease. In some people a large part of their hormone may be bound to proteins rendering them useless to our bodies. In the past taking 50mg of Zinc twice per day was what most of us in this area of medicine thought was our only option. Using zinc could result in copper depletion with increasing amounts so another option needed to be found. More research has shown that we have two additional ways to increase our levels of free testosterone. The two most commonly cited herbs for this are Avena Sativa, at 500 mg-1000 mg at breakfast along with Stinging Nettle, at 500 mg. As is the case with all neutraceuticals quality is the issue. There are some national standards that the more popular herbal neutraceuticals must achieve. You can check the United States Pharmacopeia (USP), which checks for potency and purity. As well as looking up the FDA's "Findings of Safety and Efficacy". When it comes to our health, every detail matters.

When I ask my patients what their biggest fear is when it comes to being overweight, it is usually the development of diabetes. Testosterone is a big player when administering hormones because of all that it protects the patient from, and all that it enables the patient to accomplish. In weight management, this means avoiding the onset of diabetes and the complications of this most debilitative disease, including amputation from poor circulation, kidney failure, and blindness. When testosterone is low, acquiring abdominal fat is a common occurrence especially in men. This sort of fat deposition causes heart disease, an increase in estrogen (through conversion of even the lowest amounts of testosterone to estrogen by aromatase) which can cause a drop in libido, and more seriously prostate cancer in males, insulin resistance, and all of the complications that go along with developing full blown diabetes.

If I were to throw in high triglycerides and low HDL we would have a diagnosis of "Metabolic Syndrome" or "Syndrome X". These are diagnoses no one wants to receive from their doctor. Research has shown that levels of testosterone in men above 550 ng/dl are optimal. This is especially true for ensuring that adequate levels of HDL are maintained. HDL is known as the "good" cholesterol because this molecule attaches to our "bad" cholesterol and transports it to the liver to be metabolized. This has proven to be one of the many avenues where testosterone is beneficial in the prevention of atherosclerosis and coronary artery disease.

Testosterone levels usually start to decline in the mid-thirties, and it is most likely not a coincidence that depression, the overweight/obese condition, and inflammatory disorders also begin around this age. By age 65-70, 40-50% of men have lost the ability to produce their own testosterone. Fears abound that testosterone cause's prostate cancer. This is far from the truth. Men start making this hormone in large amounts at puberty, yet the incidence of prostate cancer does not rise until they age and lose this hormone. As a matter of fact a few more correlations can be made. As testosterone levels decline men tend to gain weight in their mid-section. They gain weight because they have no energy to exercise, and also because this is a genetically predominant place for men to store fat. When they finally do get out there and exercise they get so sore and it takes so long to recover they simply give up. This is because of low testosterone levels!

Fat around the midsection is dangerous for men, as well as for women for many of the same reasons. As a matter of fact the diminished amount of testosterone older men live with is actually increasing their risk of prostate cancer. This is because the testosterone, although not enough to help maintain lean muscle and their weight is converted to estradiol by aromatase which is released by the abdominal fat which is almost impossible for these men to keep under control. The estradiol being created because of this abdominal fat substantially increases the risk of prostate cancer as previously mentioned.

Let's take a second to look at some other ways abdominal fat makes our lives so difficult. This fat that is wrapped in and around your abdominal organs puts pressure on all of the organs in the area. When we take a breath, a muscle called the diaphragm actually pulls the lungs down. This downward direction pulls the air into the lungs. When there is an increased amount of this abdominal fat, it prevents the diaphragm from fully lowering. If your diaphragm is not able to go downwards, your lungs do not fill with an appropriate amount of oxygen. Pretty tough to exercise when you cannot breathe. It is just as difficult to control asthma symptoms when an already restrictive airway is receiving less oxygen with each breath. The pressure on the liver is also another issue. All of the blood from the lower portions of our body has to pass through the center of the liver on a pathway back to the heart. The pressure of this abdominal fat on the liver, and the vein passing through it essentially creates a higher pressure gradient for the blood to flow through. This creates back pressure termed "portal pressure" which causes swelling in the legs.

As abdominal fat accumulates, and testosterone continues to get converted to estrogen and deposited in the prostate, the gland just keeps getting bigger which tends to result in urinary problems as one of the first signs of an enlarged gland. If nothing is done a small revolt will occur within the band of estrogen hormones and cancer ensues taking the owner of the prostate out of the picture. Therefore the longer that a patients' primary care doctor lets him walk around overweight, thinking foggy, and with an elevated waist to hip ratio; doing nothing about this weight or testosterone levels the MORE at risk the man is of developing prostate cancer.

I am amazed at the number of physicians still apprehensive about testosterone supplementation. This apprehension extends across the entire spectrum of prostate pathology, from an enlarged prostate to outright prostate cancer. The ridiculous fact is that the apprehension stems from the work of Huggins and Hodges that was published in 1941! Their work was important and won them the Nobel Prize. It should not be surprising that a little more research has been published over the last SEVENTY YEARS. You can help your doctor out by telling them to open up their eyes and minds and begin their enlightenment at www.testosteroneupdate.org. I do not believe a doctor could find a website easier to type into a search engine even if they did not know the name of a site to search for. "Hmmm I wonder if there has been an update on the use of testosterone over the last 70 years."

Chances are low that this will make a dent, so you need to take your health and lives into your own hands and go to places like the above site and others to become educated yourself. Research has now shown that the relationship between androgens (testosterone) and prostate cancer has changed. Well it has changed in the doctors that actually continue to read journal articles related to the disorders and patient population they treat. We now know that high testosterone levels are not synonymous with an increased chance of causing prostate cancer.

If a man has both a large abdomen and prostate, is over 50, and has a low testosterone level with all the symptoms that go along with that then he has a higher risk of developing prostate cancer than the average 170 pound healthy male. That I believe everyone can agree upon. All of the males that receive testosterone replacement at my clinic ALSO take supplements and/or a medication to protect their prostate and inhibit aromatase. I do this even though there is no proof that taking bio-identical testosterone directly causes prostate cancer. **However** I do become a bit more concerned with the scenario of a male who has a large abdomen and has more opportunity to convert supplemented testosterone to estrogen. This is because, and I cannot overstate this enough, estrogen and being overweight are the primary culprits in the development of prostate cancer, not the testosterone in and of itself. Therefore I always make sure this treatment is combined with a weight management program to quickly get rid of the abdominal fat. Testosterone in later life is a much needed hormone in both men and women to stay healthy and prevent weight gain. For men and women the weight gain in the abdomen is more dangerous than I think any of them truly understand. I will offer a few alternatives for the more conservative doctor when it comes to protecting the prostate:

Figure 8: Alternatives to Finasteride or Avodart:
- Anastrozole: 0.5-1mg twice per week
- Quercetin: 500mg-1000mg twice per day
- Curcumin: 500mg-1000mg twice per day
- Vitamin D: 5,000IU once per day
- Lycopene: 30mg once daily

This visceral fat mentioned above also releases a chemical called resistin. What is the problem with resistin? It makes the person who has a large waist circumference resistant to the effects of insulin. What is the job of insulin? Its job is to pull the sugar out of the blood and get it into the cells of our body to be used for energy. As the abdominal fat increases and the amount of resistin increases, more and more insulin is needed to rid the blood stream of sugar. This eventually takes its toll on the pancreas which results in diabetes. All of this is covered in detail in the section on diabetes.

TESTIMONIAL:

Kudos' to Dr. A:

Long before I met Dr. Ashworth I was considering having liposuction surgery on my mid section. Even though I worked out on a regular basis and had a 29 inch waistline I still could not get rid of some fat pockets. However the cost kept me from doing the procedure. I was also interested in increasing my muscle mass and raising my energy levels.

Of course the first line of thought was to do anabolic steroids. I knew of many people who did, but I preferred not to do so. When I met Dr. Ashworth and told him of my desire. He informed me of a weight management program that under his care he could design a program for me by use of bio-identical testosterone implants {which is time released into the body) and would help me improve my muscle mass, by raising my testosterone levels, and increasing my energy level. And the best part was because it wasn't anabolic steroids it would be legal and therefore under the care of a doctor. (Not in the backroom of the gym.)

I was so impressed with his knowledge, training and education on weight management that I had both procedures done. He did the testosterone implants as well as performed the liposculpting around the "Love Handle" area, and I have had great success with both.

When you talk with Dr. Ashworth you immediately know he is passionate about his work and cares for each of his patients as if they were family members. I guess in some respects we are family members sharing a common thread of self improvement. And "Dr. A", as I call him is head of the house. Like any true family member he will never advise you to do something if your best interest and health would be comprised.

I look forward to a continued relationship with Dr. A.

D H
Age 50
Weight 170
Muscle mass index 13%
AKA "Benjamin Button, 50 going on 35"

Growth Hormone:

I am always asked if I will ever start administering growth hormone. The answer right now is no. There is as much contradictory research regarding its use as there is research supporting its use. What I can say from experience is that when I am faced with a patient that is low on both growth hormone and testosterone, administering the correct amount of testosterone has yet to fail me. All of the symptoms that were ailing them, keeping them from losing the weight, and controlling weight regain were taken care of. Even more important is that I have not run into any imbalances that have occurred, because I chose testosterone over growth hormone, whether dealing with a man or a woman.

What I will do is give you a couple of supplements that are known to increase levels of growth hormone if you still retain the ability to make this hormone when stimulated to do so. The most well studied combination is Arginine at a dose of 1.2 Grams, taken along with Lysine at the same dose of 1.2 Grams which can significantly increase the production of growth hormone. High intensity exercise will also increase levels of growth hormone, and lower stress.

DHEA:

DHEA is a hormone that produces both testosterone and the estrogens. In fact, the majority of supplemented DHEA in men is converted to estrone not testosterone. This is not the case with women where DHEA will be converted to testosterone to a higher degree. The best way for men and women to get their levels of testosterone or estradiol higher is by taking the bio-identical alternative of testosterone or estradiol. It is important to understand though that low levels of DHEA have been associated with cancer, depression, auto immune disease, heart disease, and other chronic diseases. Low levels and high levels have been associated with an increased risk of breast cancer.

One of the main problems with taking DHEA without checking other hormones is that taking it first, because it is a precursor or "upstream" substrate of so many other hormones, can lower the production of other hormones from the adrenal glands that a person may need. It does this by lowering the secretion of ACTH from the brain when it senses low levels of important hormones. These hormones would have been made downstream from DHEA in normal circumstances. More than one source of information is needed to finalize a decision on any medical issue. But many people will read one article, or visit one website and decide that it must be true because of a host of reasons that in many cases make no sense what so ever.

The form of DHEA if needed is 7-keto DHEA. This is the most bioavailable and safe form of the supplement. The optimal dose is 25-100 mg per day in men, and 12.5-25mg in women. The optimal measured serum level is 400-600 micrograms/dl in men and 150-300 micrograms/dl in women. In short you should not take DHEA just because you have read or been told it is good for you. It is way too important a hormone and has too much of an impact on the hormones downstream from it. Low levels are associated with the following:

Figure 9: Symptoms of low levels of DHEA:
• Obesity
• Type II DM
• Immune Dysfunction
• Cancer
• High Blood Pressure
• Cardiovascular disease
• Depression and loss of well being
• Low libido, Erectile dysfunction
• Osteoporosis

Cortisol:

Cortisol is produced in the adrenal glands from progesterone and androstenedione. It is the body's major defense against stress, including infections and injuries. It is your body's natural anti-inflammatory hormone. Cortisol is critical for function of the immune system as well as blood sugar regulation. The best way to measure cortisol is to correlate measurements with different times of the day when optimal ranges have been determined. Having a lot of stress in your life that you are <u>not in control</u> of can cause adrenal fatigue which can definitely affect your cortisol levels. This in turn will make controlling your weight much more difficult. <u>This is discussed in</u>

more detail later in the book under Adrenal Fatigue. This will include which medication should be taken and how much.

I have included a table below that lists all of the different hormones that I regularly measure in a new patient:

Figure 10: Generic "Hormone Panel" when considering BHRT:
• LH
• FSH
• Total Estrogen, Estrone, Estriol, Estradiol
• Progesterone
• Total Testosterone & Free Testosterone
• TSH, T3, T4
• PSA
• CBC
• Sex Hormone Binding Globulin
• If you are a young male with low testosterone levels, it is a good idea to make sure prolactin levels are within normal limits to look for certain brain abnormalities.
• Some of these labs would be ordered for men and some for women and this list is not exhaustive.

TESTIMONIAL:

I am a 69 year old patient of Dr. Ashworth's. Over the past five years have benefited from many of the services he specializes in. I first went to him about my weight gain. On his weight management program I lost 26 pounds and downsized from a 14 to a 10 which I have managed to maintain since 2004. Since completing the program I have had Bio-Identical Hormone Replacement treatments which have had the largest impact on my life to date. The BHRT made me feel younger energized, and for the first time in a long time I was sleeping like a baby. I also went to him for other services like Botox, and Juvederm which I felt went right along with how much younger I felt. I am most grateful for the weight management though and the self esteem it offered, and I'm a much happier woman. I lead a very productive and meaningful life today. Thank you, Dr. Ashworth. You changed my world!

Stephanie

What should this hormone information mean . . . to you?

Having laboratory levels of these hormones means very little without someone having the ability to interpret them and apply them to general health and weight management issues. There are a few ways to administer the hormones and this is not always just an issue of convenience. Some hormones are best taken up into the blood using transdermal creams, others through a small pellet inserted into a pocket of fat in the hip. It will depend on the patient and the doctor, and deciding the best way to adjust the hormones as you and your doctor travel along the road back to health.

It is important to measure the hormones in a window of 6-8 weeks after initiating the first treatment. This lab level is interpreted along with how you are feeling physically and mentally. After this the levels can be measured every 5-6 months if you continue to feel well. If not then your doctor will adjust the hormone dose that would best correct how you feel, then redraw an additional lab test after 8 weeks. Another extremely important point to readdress is the delivery system for the hormones. Is the transdermal cream and pellet insertion that much better than taking a pill? The key word when dealing with a cream is "liposomal", having a liposomal delivery system is critical. It is probably one of the biggest reasons over the counter creams fail to make it into the blood stream. A liposomal drug delivery system renders the hormone both lipophilic and hydrophilic. These terms simply mean that the delivery vehicle will enable the cream to make it into your cells that are two layers thick referred to as a lipid bi-layer. So the cream must be able to mix with fat and water. It is no secret that water and oil do not mix.

So making a cream that is able to deal with both is pretty unique. Another important point is that the cream needs to be ready to be attacked by our body. When these liposomal delivery systems are created correctly they incorporate a protective layer against immune destruction by the body. All of the transdermal creams we carry at our clinic are delivered through a liposomal delivery system, and are delivered to us from a very reputable compounding pharmacy.

The lesson to be learned in regards to BHRT is to bring your body back to a place where you had control over how you dealt with daily life, stress, exercise, not just calories. It is about taking out some of the guess work from aging and how you are supposed to feel as you age. This is not just the case with using the hormones for what I have mentioned as it relates to reducing weight. It also applies to the ability of your skin to make and retain collagen and elastin! What is it about younger women that make their skin so beautiful, smooth, and tight? It is the availability of hormones!

The take home point is that you do have a choice. You don't have to just wonder off into the sunset as an apple shaped diabetic with a headache caused by high blood pressure. The good news is there is a healthy choice when looking at replacement of hormones. If a clinic that concentrates on weight management does not also deal with the issue of declining hormones; then this clinic is not fully equipped to help in your weight management efforts and especially in your weight management maintenance. Many clinics, both medical and non-medical, as well as some of the over the counter pills sold in health food stores can help you lose weight, but there are very few that help you keep it off once you are done. There are many that end up harming you in a way that may make it nearly impossible to keep the weight off for any significant period of time. What is this "period of time to keep the weight off" . . . as far as I am concerned you need to keep the weight off the rest of your life!

Before closing out this section I want to make one thing clear, certain situations warrant caution and patience. If a woman walks into my clinic and she has a history of breast cancer and it was estrogen or progesterone positive cancer she will not be put on hormones of any kind. We do however need to make sure any and all additional disorders are treated. Like I have written previously, prior to the use of HRT it wasn't that the women I was noticing having trouble losing weight did not lose any weight at all, they were just losing it slower than the 3-5 pounds I like to see each week. Many women are just happy to see consistent weight coming off every week. This is whether it is 2 pounds or 5 pounds! The point is they are finally reducing weight WITHOUT losing muscle. When we have a hormone situation that is not able to be treated because of safety reasons, we just need to address everything that can be treated safely, and be more vigilant with the exercise and keep the cheating episodes to a minimum.

That is the key though. If something like declining hormones is beyond your ability to have treated, then the life after weight management will be a strict one. But will it be worth it? Of course it will. I would never send a woman off into the maintenance phase empty handed. She always has all of the tools necessary to keep the weight off. I am used to being the" last ditch guy". This is whether a woman has a uterus and ovaries and makes plenty of hormones or not, the job gets done! There's more than one way to increase a metabolic rate and a person's ability to burn fat. It just takes some tricks of the trade and that requires having done "the trade" for a while, which I have and which this book will show.

Knowledge is power! My job is to take all the time needed to make sure every patient knows and understands why I do what I do to help them lose weight. There may be a time in their life when I am not available because they have moved. But at least they have all of the knowledge regarding the appropriate types of foods, how to exercise, the importance of water and certain nutrients. This will get them through whatever it is they are challenged with. We will always have to continue eating. Food is not like alcohol or other drugs where you can just stop cold turkey. You will always have to continue to eat and control the relationship you have with food both psychologically and physically. Having a firm grip on how and why the body handles calories is powerful knowledge.

> **_POW:_ _IF THERE EVER WAS A SECRET TO WEIGHT LOSS OVER 40, OR A FOUNTAIN OF YOUTH, BIO-IDENTICAL HRT IS BOTH!_**

CHAPTER 6

Are you suffering from Adrenal Fatigue?

Being "Stressed Out" is likely the most common complaint proclaimed by the general public. What do we associate with being "Stressed Out"? The first condition that most of us would answer with is Adrenal Fatigue. We need to look at some serious adrenal conditions at first and then progress to more common causes of adrenal fatigue. Is this a case of Addison's disease, where all of the hormones normally secreted by the adrenals are low to non-existent (not likely but possible)? Or is this a dysfunction due to adrenal burnout secondary to high stress, chronic illness, high carbohydrate intake, alcohol, or other toxins taken on a regular basis? Do you have any idea how many people walk into my clinic and say they are absolutely addicted to carbohydrates? I can tell you it is a lot and that carbohydrates can be very addictive. Later in the book under the nutrition section I write about specific foods that are addictive and why. The most common reason for adrenal fatigue in those 40 years old and above, is simply an age related reduction in the adrenal glands ability to produce enough hormones. This occurs primarily when the ovaries and testicles begin to slow down and we begin to rely more and more on the adrenal glands. Because remember the adrenals secrete every hormone the testicles and ovaries secrete plus some.

Some other conditions that interfere with adrenal function are very serious viral infections that are prolonged like chronic fatigue syndrome and the myriad of conditions this syndrome can be responsible for. Another is a discontinuation of high dose corticosteroid therapy. When the adrenals are subjected to high dose outside sources of corticosteroids like <u>prednisone</u>, they will stop normal production of the adrenal hormones you are accustomed to. When that outside source is abruptly discontinued the body is basically left with nothing for a while—at least until the adrenals start to pick up production of cortisol if able to do so at all.

Figure 11: Common Symptoms of Adrenal Fatigue
- Many of the same symptoms as an inactive thyroid
- Increased pigmentation (discoloration of the skin)
- Weakness
- Hypotension (low blood pressure)
- Gastrointestinal disturbances (abdominal pain, diarrhea, constipation)
- Episodes of low blood sugar
- Salt cravings
- In females, there may be a loss of under arm hair and pubic hair
- Inability to recover from mild, common cold symptoms

Most jobs where people find themselves developing adrenal fatigue are the ones where they feel as though they have little control over their lives. The fact is that many people simply eat more food when they are stressed. A couple of the main hormones that are released during times of stress are DHEA and Cortisol (which is no surprise). The interesting point regarding cortisol levels is that, as most of our other hormones in our body are decreasing, cortisol is actually one that <u>increases</u> with age. This is sort of the problem also. The lives that I describe, full of stress and pressure are what fatigue our adrenal glands. Most of this occurs when we are younger in our "prime" working our tail ends off, all the while draining these important glands of their ability to take care of us when we get older. Hasn't someone said we are supposed to have "Golden Years" when we retire (if we retire)? It seems as though I hear more people right in the middle of these supposed golden years making cynical jokes and negative comments when they are smack in the middle of these great years.

When people are stressed, they are also releasing epinephrine. This hormone can actually make us feel good, and some people get addicted to that feeling. This is one reason why people may say "I handle stress well." They just may not realize how harmful stress can be. When or if we ever get a serious disease, we need our adrenals to be in good rested, working order to help fight off the ailment. People with Chronic Fatigue Syndrome need to have their adrenals looked at. Just as that disorder's name tells us, it is a chronic condition that completely drains the person suffering from it

An accurate way to test for insufficient adrenal glands is to take four saliva samples at differing times throughout the day. These are times of the day where in general we know what the levels should look like, and this will give us a good idea if there is a problem with production. This is a test result where you and the doctor need to discuss the results together. You do not want to be in the low-normal range and have the doctor tell you it is normal. Remember the doctor needs to be treating you and the lab levels. You also want to look for levels that seem to go way up then drop way down; because this is not good and whether you are low, low-normal, or at the extremes of high and low, treatment needs to be initiated when these levels are in combination with physical symptoms.

A very interesting occurrence begins to take place if this condition goes untreated. The body will actually begin to break down progesterone, which cortisol is made from. This will lead to over-abundance or an out of balance sex hormone situation between progesterone, estrogen, and testosterone. We desperately need all of our hormones in balance, and the cortisol deficiency needs to be dealt with as soon as possible. Since progesterone is our calming hormone, and the body is breaking down too much of it, sleeping soundly will become a thing of the past. If a female's estrogen levels begin to dominate, she may start to notice prolonged menstruation with heavy bleeding. If this is not treated, repeated heavy menstrual cycles that her body is not accustomed to dealing with could lead to an anemic state. The problems then really begin to pile up that need to be dealt with.

The following is another great patient example. I saw a 50 year old woman that had the classic signs of adrenal fatigue and low hormones in general. She mentioned an episode where she had been running herself ragged 2 years prior. She had not menstruated since having her one and only child in her mid forties. As most of us, she was trying to make ends meet and was not sleeping well and working 6 days per week. She had little control over her work schedule and began to find herself getting increasingly more tired as each day passed. It began to get harder to get the work done in the allotted time because her fatigue was getting worse. The next thing she knew was that she woke up in an ambulance, having had a seizure lasting 4 minutes. The adrenals are responsible for our electrolytes, like salt and potassium. In medical school we would say the adrenals are responsible for sugar, salt, and sex. Even though she was menopausal she had not been having a lot of the symptoms of menopause prior to this because the adrenals can produce the same hormones as the ovaries. She pushed her adrenals to the limit and beyond. She was referred to me to fix her hormones. The amazing part of the 6 days she spent in the ICU was that one of her major medications was an anti-anxiety medication by IV that kept her sleeping, thereby giving the adrenal glands a much needed break.

Adrenal Fatigue Patient Example:

It is incredible when what I write about plays out so clearly in the clinic. The most recent was a patient that had been trying to get her thyroid "straightened out" for 5 years by a range of other physician specialists! The treatment for low adrenal function and hypothyroidism go hand in hand. Trying to treat the thyroid without addressing the adrenal glands can, at times, lead to a dead end. If you have been at an optimum dose of thyroid medicine for a long time and then start to feel like you did previously, instead of immediately jumping into more thyroid tests and an increased dose ask your doctor to take a look at the adrenals. When I write to look at the adrenals I am not just referring to cortisol. I am referring to all of the sex hormones as well, testosterone, estradiol, and progesterone. People may begin to <u>feel worse</u> after starting their thyroid medication if there is a problem with the adrenals. The woman I am referring to had been put on Synthroid and the labs that were ordered to check the effectiveness of the dose she was on was missing a critical value, a T3. This lab value actually represents the most important hormone the thyroid produces, and the primary hormone the body responds to. If this hormone level is so important why was it not ordered by the fine doctor who placed her on Synthroid? That is an excellent question and will be covered in detail in the chapter covering Hypothyroidism. I feel compelled to mention at this point that I have never written a prescription for Synthroid in a person I diagnosed with Hypothyroidism, and again I will explain why in more detail in the Thyroid section. But suffice it to say that it in my opinion it has never been the effectiveness of Synthroid that has made it such a commonly written prescription for hypothyroidism, it has more to do with the effectiveness of the company's marketing campaign. Before getting carried away in the wrong chapter I will step down from the soap box now and get back to the patient I was discussing. She was not on any other hormone replacement aside from Synthroid, had not had any other hormonal levels tested; and a lot of her symptoms seemed to mimic being low on one or all of the top three sex hormones: estradiol, progesterone, and testosterone.

The first order of business was to switch her over to Armour Thyroid, which I prefer because of a number of reasons yet to be discussed. I then sent her for additional labs. This patient was in her late twenties and frankly I did not feel as though her adrenal glands could be fatigued at such an early time in her life. Because she had been on the birth control pill for many years her sex hormone levels were way out of balance so I started her on very low doses of a couple of the bio-identical hormones she was in need of getting balanced. She admitted that she felt "a little better" but most of her symptoms remained after over 6 weeks! There it was right in front of me, a classic adrenal fatigue patient. I put her on Cortef 10 mg per day spread throughout the day, and as I anticipated everything started to turn around and respond as expected. She eventually was able to discontinue the Cortef and when she stopped taking the pill she was able to enjoy her natural hormone levels as her ovaries kicked back in. This was yet another testament to all of the hormones needing to be in balance, and the thyroid not responding to appropriate treatment without the adrenal glands being taken care of. I think it should also prove that making these diagnoses are not easy and can take time.

How to Treat Adrenal Fatigue:

Deciding on the best treatment option can be a tough decision. Natural therapies are always the best to try first. The first most conservative approach prior to things getting really bad is to take a vacation and get rid of the stress in your life allowing your adrenals rest. If that just is not enough, then there are raw glandular capsules that can be taken. The problems with these are that they come from cattle and contamination may be an issue. The other major problem is that these medicines are designed to force the adrenals to make more cortisol. This in turn will just wear out the adrenal glands, in the same manner that some diabetic medicines affect the pancreas, by forcing it to make more insulin. If any raw glandular capsules are taken, it has been written that the New Zealand Glandular is the best.

An appropriate diet is crucial when dealing with adrenal issues. This should come as no surprise since in essence we are what we eat. Specifically, for the adrenals, a program with appropriate amounts of protein is critical. You should also eat every 3-4 hours, if possible, or 5 small meals throughout the day. It is always helpful to cut back on any carbohydrate loading and increase the intake of low glycemic index fruits and especially vegetables. High sugar foods and highly refined carbohydrates need to be avoided. These types of foods are in and of themselves stressful to the adrenal glands. Stressed adrenals are also unable to handle extremely high protein diets. So Atkins sort of programs are out of the question. We need to concentrate on well-balanced, low GI carbohydrates, with "good" fats and normal amounts of bio-available protein. Being hungry all the time should also be avoided. I strive to make sure that all of my patients do not walk around hungry. Salt treatment should be liberalized, especially in the cases of patients that consistently show up with low blood pressures, meaning below 100/60. Why salt when we are told that salt needs to be avoided in order to control blood pressure? There are a couple of reasons for this thinking. Remember, the adrenals are responsible for sugar, salt, and sex. It is the salt portion of this three pronged secretion I focus on. I will run labs and check the patients' electrolytes and adrenal function prior to initiating any treatment. When people are on a weight management program they are usually encouraged to drink plenty of water. Many people take this to the extreme and drink much more than the 64 ounces required. In some individuals this amount of water begins to dilute the blood. This can have an effect on blood pressure by actually lowering it to the point of light headedness. If a patient is not on high blood pressure medicines I will usually advise that they add a small amount of salt to their foods. If this helps then we have the diagnosis. If not then I need to dig further and find out the cause.

Adjusting hormone levels with bio-identical hormones is also an option. If a woman is low in progesterone, the hormone that makes cortisol, this hormone can be given which can boost the levels of cortisol. As a side note progesterone receptors are also found on the thyroid! This is all interconnected and if ANYONE thinks they can handle weight management without being able to handle a person's hormones they are nuts. Keep in mind that when you take something like progesterone you also need to balance out estradiol, especially if dealing with a post-menopausal person. As with everything else I have written about, the first place to get a definitive diagnosis is to test the blood or urine. So once the levels of cortisol are tested there are a few directions we can go in depending on whether it is high or low.

Figure 12: Test level of Cortisol:

If they are high:

- Lifestyle changes are in order in an effort to eliminate stress when possible
- Meditation

If they are low:

- Adrenal support: as discussed below using vitamins, minerals, or as above glandular
- You can also take over-the-counter vitamins and nutrients. Chromium is a vital nutrient. It is a great supplement for increasing insulin sensitivity and decreasing sugar cravings. An aging adrenal gland carries less and less chromium. It can be taken at a standard daily dose of 400 mg/day
- Licorice Root is good for the adrenals when they are stressed and trying to recover. Start at 2-3 grams/ twice each day for 6 weeks, then taper down by taking it once every other day for 2 weeks, then just for two days the third week
- You can also take Pantothenic Acid 200 mg twice per day till the adrenals start to feel like they are recovering and your energy is improving
- Any good vitamin store should have a mixture of Tocopherols, which are organic compounds that are essentially fat-soluble antioxidants—Vitamin A, which is a fat-soluble vitamin, can be taken at 40,000 IU daily. These fat-soluble vitamins need to be taken with caution. They can accumulate in our bodies and become toxic. Recent research has also advised against supplementation with Vitamin E because of adverse effects on the cardiovascular system. Lastly vitamin B6 can be taken at 50 mg daily and B12 at 1000 mcg daily until the adrenals recover.
- Concentrate on rest and plenty of sleep

Figure 13: Symptoms of Cortisol deficiency:
- Fatigue
- Anxiety, nervousness
- Poor stress tolerance
- Hypersensitivity to environment
- Absent-minded, forgetful, feeling spacey and easily confused
- Depression
- Paranoid
- Irritable, hostile
- Concentration problems

How do we know when the adrenals have recovered?

Once you start to feel more energy and the symptoms listed begin improving, then you again take the appropriate test that gives the most accurate results and find out. It is best to use the same lab at which the original lab values were attained. This way a comparison can be made. Of course, when the adrenals are healthy you will begin to drop weight easier.

Natural therapies like the ones listed previously are always the best to try first. Although when I tell a person to take a vacation or to try and simply relax more, they look at me like I am a nut case. When these fail, or when the person continues to sit there looking at me like I'm a nut case until I offer a "more realistic treatment", a more aggressive approach will be needed. This more aggressive approach is the use of hydrocortisone. The doses advocated have been used for years and are 10-20 mg/day. This dosing has not been associated with any negative side effects or known to have caused the adrenals to stop making hormone naturally. The latter side effect is not likely when one considers that the reason I am starting the hydrocortisone is because the adrenals are fatigued and not secreting enough. The absolute best way to approach this dosage is to split the 20 mg into 4 doses at 5mg each spread throughout the day. When taking the hydrocortisone in this way it will help you realize why, at certain points in history, this medication has been considered a miracle drug! The type of hydrocortisone I am referring to is called Cortef, and another is Hysone-4 these being as close to mimicking natural cortisol as possible. Some people are born with slow acting adrenals and require treatment early on in life. It is not unreasonable for them to stay on the medicine long term as long as the dose is kept low.

Since the book is written in the hopes of helping people help their doctor integrate weight management into their practice, it would be prudent to mention the commonly known side-effect of taking this medicine-hunger. Why is hunger experienced? It has been postulated that in patients where the cortisol levels have been chronically low, there have most likely been associated gastrointestinal problems that has lead to poor absorption of nutrients. Once treatment is started and in an effort to quickly replenish these nutrients the body's response is to trigger eating. Some patients simply get hungry, and I firmly believe that cortisol stimulates the hunger center in the brain. The truth is most people report that this stage only lasts 2-3 weeks then subsides. The physician administering the hydrocortisone should be ready for this and should be there to help the patient get through it so that this side effect is dealt with.

In patients that cannot seem to produce their own Cortisol, make sure your doctor includes an ACTH lab level, the cortisol stimulating hormone from the brain. When dealing with the adrenals, the other hormones that the adrenal gland produces cannot be ignored. Therefore, measure DHEA levels and especially aldosterone. Aldosterone helps to control the levels of electrolytes in our bodies, like potassium and salt. **DHEA is the hormone that all three estrogens and testosterone are made from so its importance cannot be overstated.** If tests find that DHEA is low, it needs to be taken as 7-keto DHEA. The dose is usually 25 mg/day. This will cut down on masculinization effects such as acne and facial hair in women when this supplement is at higher doses. There are those that take DHEA like it was a simple vitamin. This is not the way to look at this supplement, or any supplement for that matter; especially supplements that are directly involved in the production of vital hormones. When DHEA is taken the body's natural production of it will diminish, and so will the natural downstream hormones that are normally produced! This is a vital point especially if you are the sort that forgets to take their supplements. In other words, your body starts to rely on this outside source of DHEA to use in the production of those other vital hormones. When you stop taking that outside source, and your natural production, as minimal as it may have been also has diminished, you will be sitting in a position much worse than you were previously.

In the end, if there is no serious medical condition and your adrenals retain some production capability, the way to bring the adrenals back to good working order is to decrease how much stress you are exposed to and how you learn to deal with that stress. Just from this section on adrenal fatigue, you should be able to see that treating a person who is overweight is no easy task. Therefore, it is not a surprise that so many fail in their attempts to lose weight. Just keep your heads up and take your healthcare into your hands by encouraging your doctor to do all he or she can do to make sure that all bases are covered. I do not expect nor advise anyone to self treat. This book is meant to provide the reader the knowledge they need to open up lines of communication with your doctor as to how they can approach helping you lose weight.

If you feel unusually tired over a long period of time, do not let anyone tell you not to worry. Always believe that you know your body better than anyone else, because you do. Take the time to look through all of the symptoms represented in this book. It is important to do your own due diligence when it comes to your health care. Nobody outside of you and your family care as much about your health. There are lazy people out there responsible for some very important aspects of our lives and doctors are not immune to this. The next disorder I am writing about is very important; not because of making the diagnosis, but in how the medical community treats it.

> *POW:* *YOUR ADRENALS MAKE EVERY HORMONE THE OVARIES AND TESTICLES MAKE. THE ADRENALS ARE SUPPOSED TO KEEP YOU FEELING NORMAL LONG AFTER THOSE OTHER TWO WEAR OUT.*

CHAPTER 7

Is there a problem with your Thyroid?

In the **current medical establishment**, there are usually two issues that come to mind when someone has an unexplained weight gain. First, the person is simply eating too much and not getting enough exercise. Second, there must be something wrong with their thyroid. There will be doctors out there that will tell you an underactive thyroid will not cause weight gain. This is completely untrue; *of course* an underactive thyroid can cause weight gain. If you were walking around with a decreased metabolic rate, sluggish, unable to concentrate, had a grayish hue, swelling around the eyes, extremely fatigued, depressed, constipated, and picked as an extra in a zombie movie with no audition you also would be convinced that the thyroid is an important issue in overall health and weight management. If the thyroid was treated appropriately and all of those symptoms resolved, and the person started to lose weight, I would be very compelled to say the thyroid had a lot to do with weight gain. Just because the medicine my colleagues continue to use does not result in weight loss, does not mean that hypothyroidism is unrelated to weight gain. In reality when this medication, that I will introduce you to, is used in the treatment of hypothyroidism the reason no weight loss is seen is because they have done little to nothing for the thyroid condition to begin with.

I have heard more than just one physician say that if the patient's metabolic rate is normal and their thyroid is _normal by their standards,_ the person must refuse to exercise and eat too much. All of the multitude and complex mechanisms by which the thyroid gland exerts its effects are not completely understood. However, we do know that hormones released by the thyroid <u>enhance</u> <u>oxygen consumption of most tissues of the body and is known</u> <u>to increase the basal metabolic rate</u> as well as the breakdown of carbohydrates, lipids, and proteins. Therefore, it would seem that having this gland in good working order is vitally important in any battle of the overweight condition.

TSH, T4 and T3; When getting two out of three IS BAD:

The hormone that is released in the largest amount from the thyroid is Thyroxine (T4). When the thyroid releases less than normal levels of T4, this is one major indicator of hypothyroidism. It is well known that T4 is poorly absorbed from the intestines when taken orally. A number of factors can make it difficult for the T4 to make it out of the gut; for instance abnormal intestinal bacteria, including plasma proteins, and soluble (foods that soak up water in the intestines) dietary factors. The percent of T4 absorbed from the gut is discussed in a little more detail below. This just says that you should take your thyroid medication on an empty stomach and separate from other medicines to give it the best chance of getting into your blood stream. It is important to separate taking this medication from other medications by at least 2 hours. As of the writing of this book I have yet to find a form of T4 by itself that works in the treatment of hypothyroidism. Yes, I have looked heavily into the use of Synthroid and Levoxyl and have found both to be equally useless. From this point on they will be referred to simply as T4.

Clinical experience has shown me that a low metabolic rate and hypothyroidism are intricately linked and may just be the beginning of finding out what is causing weight gain. If an underactive thyroid gland is suspected as a cause of weight gain, one of the first lab tests to order would be a Thyroid Stimulating Hormone (TSH). The best place to start is to give an explanation as to what the TSH represents. It is important that everyone understands what their doctor is trying to treat and what you should come to expect by their treatment protocols. TSH is a hormone that is released by the brain to <u>STIMULATE the thyroid to work</u>. Therefore, TSH levels **are**

high when a thyroid is **not functioning properly**, because it is as if the brain is simply yelling louder and louder at the thyroid to work. So, the *higher* the TSH, *the less* your thyroid gland is functioning. The brain knows this because the blood flows through the brain and it gets the signal that there is not enough thyroid hormone floating in the blood. So it sends out the THYROID STIMULATING HORMONE or TSH. The more it sends out, or the higher the TSH is, the less healthy the thyroid gland is.

A smart doctor realizes from the very start that this is a sign that at the very least two more tests need to be ordered to zero in on exactly what is wrong with the thyroid, and that this may indeed be the answer to the patients' weight gain. In other words when a patient keeps gaining weight and continues to complain that his or her thyroid may still be out of whack, instead of ignoring the patient it may be that something crucial is being overlooked. Those additional tests would need to include the T3!!! A trend has been gaining momentum over the last 5 years. This trend is where my colleagues are omitting a T3 from thyroid panels. When I was in medical school, the rule was to order at a minimum, all three of these lab values. This will be covered in a few paragraphs to come.

Figure 14: Symptoms of Hypothyroidism
(Personally I think all of these would make weight management tough! This is why I continue to argue that the thyroid when not functioning properly DOES cause weight gain.)

- Low temperature in the A.M.
- Minor illnesses are slow to resolve
- Decreased sweating
- Cold intolerance, dry skin
- Lateral thinning of the eyebrows; swollen eyelids, tongue & hands
- Resistance to weight management
- Fatigue, sluggish, concentration difficulties, memory loss, depression
- On the flip side, anxiety and agitation (at soccer games), although nonspecific, can be a signal of hypothyroidism
- Constipation, bloating
- Feet and leg cramps at night

Additional details of Hypothyroidism:

Remember, it is called hypothyroid or having an underactive thyroid, but the TSH will be high, not low. Recall that the TSH is trying to get your thyroid gland to make more thyroid hormone because you have a poorly performing thyroid gland.

The intensity of these symptoms will typically be more pronounced in the morning (except for feet and leg cramps at night) or at rest and will be spread all over the body. Having all or even just a couple of the more serious of the above symptoms alone is enough to cause weight gain. It may be true that hypothyroidism does not actually turn a protein into a fat, but it definitely makes it easier for the calories you take in to end up being stored as fat in your body! It is also worth mentioning that it has been well studied that thyroid hormones modulate or in simpler terms is able to adjust and control the amount of carbohydrates, fat, and protein in our bodies. I mention this because some physicians seem to love to say, "Hypothyroidism does not make you fat". Well, it sure does not help a person live lean! Furthermore they need to keep their opinions to themselves until they start ordering the appropriate lab values that guide diagnosis and treatment. The symptoms listed above can be so profound that just getting out of bed can be a struggle. So I say, yes, hypothyroidism can and does lead to weight gain if this gland and its hormones are not treated appropriately. So to all that disagree with that morsel of controversial information they can take it home and chew on it, it's yummy.

Without a properly operating thyroid, or at least an adequate amount of a useable form of thyroid floating through the blood stream, an attempt at weight management does not make much of a difference in the long run. The long run is what we are after because in weight management medicine "The means need to justify the end". Once you lose the initial weight, you never want to gain more than five to ten pounds again without asking yourself why. I tell my patients when five to ten pounds return, it is time to come back in and make sure everything is still on track. We want to address all of the issues that will make weight maintenance possible. I could care less about adding up all of the pounds of fat that I have helped patient's lose over the years. What I do care about is the number of people that have not gained the weight back after losing all of that weight.

Figure 15: Causes of Hypothyroidism

Primary Hypothyroidism: (95% of cases)
- Idiopathic (In other words, we really do not know why the thyroid quit working)
- Hashimotos Thyroiditis (test for this by having your doctor test for thyroid peroxidase antibodies)
- Irradiation secondary to Thyroiditis
- Graves Disease
- Surgical Removal
- Fibrous Thyroiditis Late Stage
- Iodine Deficiency
- Drug Therapy (Lithium, Interferon)
- Infiltrative Diseases (Sarcoidosis, Amyloidosis, Scleroderma, Hemochromatosis)

Secondary Hypothyroidism: (5% of cases)
- Cancer of Pituitary
- Cancer of Hypothalamus
- Congenital Hypopituitarism
- Pituitary Necrosis (Sheehan's syndrome)
- Adrenal Insufficiency

What is a normal TSH level?

The answer will vary from doctor to doctor, and you as the patient need to take control of your health. The most recent literature is that a TSH level below 2.0 is adequate. The problem occurs when your average level over the last 20 years may have been 0.75 (which is below 2.0), BUT when accompanied by weight gain and other symptoms of hypothyroidism listed previously, should alert the doctor to do a more thorough investigation. The basic rule of labs is never just treating a lab value. Treat the lab value in concert with how the patient feels at that particular value. I have patients whose lab values may indicate they are taking an "adequate" dosage of thyroid medication, but my patient does not feel "adequate"; therefore I may opt for more thyroid medication in an effort to help my patient feel their best. Safety, of course, always comes first, so I pay strict attention to all of the indications of taking too much of any and all medications. But in the end, all people are different. What might work for one person may not work for the next, so physicians need to be flexible and ready to think outside of the standard medical box. Above average treatment is what my patients have come to expect from me and what you should expect from your doctor.

The other two lab values that you, as the patient, need to understand are what T4 and Thyronine (T3) levels mean. The body uses the <u>ACTIVE</u> thyroid hormone T3 by primarily <u>converting it</u> from T4. "Active" meaning that T3 is the hormone that helps you feel and function at your best. T3 is actually four times as strong as T4. T3 is also bound to less protein when it is floating in the blood stream, which renders it more metabolically available than T4. T3 is 8 to 10 times more available as a free unbound hormone than T4. Only about 0.03% of T4 is available once it starts circulating in the blood. Let us look at T4 and T3 as two fighters in the ring. T4 is a big popular fighter, but not because he is better than T3 he is just better known and has a lot of sponsors . . . . like big pharmaceutical companies. T3 is by far the better fighter, but comes from a smaller gym with less money for sponsoring and building a strong brand for the fighter. People who have been around the game long enough know that T3 will perform much better than T4. When T3 steps into the ring with the over rated T4, a good old fashioned, passionate butt whooping occurs. In the end it is T3 that is the winner hands down, every time.

The heart has no way, on its own, to convert T4 to T3, and, yes, it requires T3 to function properly. There are very popular medications on the market *that are only formulated as T4*. Your body is then supposed to convert that T4 to T3, which occurs primarily in the liver. There are problems I want to mention with using medications that are only formulated as T4. These problems are centered on how T4 and T3 do their jobs, or more specifically having an environment where they can do their jobs unhindered. Below I listed a few of the many problems that I have with how standard medicine approaches the treatment of this vital gland:

1. You may not be able to convert T4 to T3 in your body. The medication you are taking may simply be unable to be converted to the more active T3 (This is the most likely cause with the medications most commonly prescribed). It is not so important that you know all of the reasons why this is the case, that is your doctor's problem. It is just important that he or she knows that *you know conversion* may be a concern that needs addressing. You ask if the medicine he or she just prescribed for your hypothyroidism is all T4 and to explain to you how well that medicine converts to T3. Then just wait a few moments and stare at them, waiting for a "conversion" explanation and what they are going to do about it.

2. Certain medications that you take make it very difficult for your body to utilize your thyroid medicine if it is only coming in the form of T4, so ask. Remember T4 is not the big player, T3 is. Propanolol, a beta-blocker high blood pressure medication, can inhibit the conversion of T4 to T3. Medications like glucocortocoids (steroids) may also do this. If you are taking any of these types of medications (as well as those listed below), make your doctor aware that you understand that your thyroid medicine may not work very well; therefore, the dose of your thyroid medicine may need to be increased or, better yet, completely changed. (That statement is making a lot of other doctor's wince in pain because they know you may be about to mention a certain medication, first lettering of first word A, second letter of second word T.) Again simply stare, they will need to check your medication list. If they don't start to check your medication list then ask them to. I mean they are *your* medications. If something needs to be changed they will not know unless they start investigating interactions.

3. Chronic caloric deprivation, which I have seen in younger women who have a history of modeling or other occupations where an extremely low weight is smiled upon, may acquire problems with their intestinal system and subsequently acquire problems getting the thyroid medicines through the gut wall. Even in the general population, and best case scenarios T4 gets absorbed from the intestines poorly-ranging from 40-79%. On the other hand, T3 is absorbed at around 95% in 4 hours. This brings us back to the last two sentences of #2 above—the one about changing medications, doctors wincing in pain, and a lot of staring. Why so many doctors dislike the medication known as Armour Thyroid is bewildering and confusing to me. Mainly because the alternative they love prescribing is so lousy at getting the job done.

4. When chronic caloric deprivation (listed above) or anorexia nervosa is combined with liver disease, kidney failure, surgical stress, or chronic illness, it has been called "T3 Thyronine Syndrome". In other words, your thyroid medication is not making it any further than your toilet water. The study conducted for these findings took place at one hundred fashion model runway shows across the globe from Paris to New York, where teaching assistants were required to retrieve samples from the top models private portal potties. No wonder undergraduate teaching assistants are in such a bad mood all the time.

5. As we age, we *decrease* the number of receptors that pull the T4 and T3 out of our blood stream. The brain is able to monitor the amount of thyroid hormone in your blood, but does not measure the amount of available receptors in your body that can pull the thyroid hormone out of the blood stream and put it to work. So again, the labs may say everything is OK, but you still feel terrible and are exhibiting the symptoms of hypothyroidism. You may need a higher dose of thyroid medication. So what do you want your doctor to know? That a higher dose may be indicated if the T4 is coming up low, but the TSH is showing up normal on

the lab panels. In a case like this, make sure your doctor orders another set of labs where a "free" T4 and T3 are looked at prior to medication adjustments. "Free" meaning not being bound to proteins in the blood. You can measure your temperature religiously in the AM to see if the dose of thyroid medicine is working and coinciding with how you are feeling. If you are feeling better and your temperature is also normalizing, then you are probably at a good dose.

6. This next fact is simply another testament for keeping your hormones in balance. It is a proven fact that there are progesterone receptors on the thyroid gland! Therefore some people may need progesterone replacement therapy to get their thyroid working properly. Seen more often in females, and if this is the case it will be evident because the women will have low levels of progesterone, may be in menopause and all factors will be pointing the doctor in the correct direction if he or she has the proper road map.

7. I will list yet another example how only measuring the TSH and T4 leads to terrible medical care. I have witnessed firsthand a physician place their patient on a medicine such as Synthroid and continue to only check the above two labs in a futile attempt to make dosing adjustments. They see a T4 that is high normal and a TSH that has dropped to below 0.5, did not bother with a T3 or physical exam and claim their patient had hyper-Thyroidism! TSH is a stimulatory hormone. If there is nothing to stimulate then why worry about it being too low? If however the physician was to measure a T3, find it elevated and correlate this finding with a rapid heart rate or unexplained weight loss, then I would agree.

Of the issues listed above, the age issue can be the most confusing to understand. Your brain senses that the level of thyroid hormone in your blood is high and the thyroid gland does not need to be stimulated. The brain then sends out less TSH into your blood, because the brain does not think that TSH or any stimulating is necessary. So your TSH will show up on labs as low, but, in reality, what is really happening is you simply cannot use a large portion of the T3 and T4 because of a lack of receptors secondary to simply growing older. This holds true regardless of which medication your doctor uses to treat the thyroid. So in this case you may need more medication flowing through your blood stream which increases the chance of all of the available receptors being found and stimulated.

All of this comes down to basic "Being a Good Doctor 101"—treat the patient, not just the lab values. Let us revisit the nasty T3 trend that is emerging. This trend is a total disregard in the importance of ordering a T3 lab value. Sort of odd since T3 is actually the work horse of the thyroid. *Make sure your doctor measures the TSH, T4, and T3 values* at the very least, and, of course, understands how to interpret and treat. If they tell you the T3 is not necessary to evaluate simply revisit the determined blank stare that essentially says: wrong answer. They also need to be paying attention to the possibility that you may have built up antibodies that are attaching to your hormones rendering them useless. To address this with your doctor simply say: "Antibodies, I hear antibodies could be a problem how about we measure those".

> *POW: IN MY 10 + YEARS OF MEDICAL WEIGHT MANAGEMENT I HAVE NEVER FOUND SYNTHROID OR LEVOXYL TO BE EFFECTIVE. UNTIL SOMETHING BETTER COMES ALONG I HAVE AND WILL CONTINUE TO USE ARMOUR THYROID.*

A Thyroid patient example:

Patient was a 30 year old female working on her PhD seeking guidance on weight management. She was also an assistant principal with children of her own. Her stress levels were extremely high. Her resting metabolic rate when measured at our clinic actually covered up the word slow. She had a prior diagnosis of anemia and was being treated for that by her primary care doctor. This had not helped her weight management efforts (although in some instances this is definitely the problem). Her thyroid lab tests showed a normal TSH and an elevated T4. However her T3 level was below normal. Since most thyroid panels these days fail to have a T3 level ordered this undoubtedly would have been missed. Actually it was missed because in the quest to find out why she was so tired, instead of continuing to properly treat the thyroid by checking a T3, the doctor ordered an anemia profile and steered treatment in that direction. In this person it wasn't the wrong medication that was causing the problem, it was an inability to convert her natural levels of T4 to T3. But as we can see if the thyroid is left inadequately treated, it has such a huge part to play in our well being that we will continue to suffer. As physicians we need to get back to ordering a complete thyroid panel!!! The next endocrinology meeting I attend I am going to wear a T-shirt that has "Order a T3 on all of your hypothyroid patients!" just to drive home that point.

As mentioned previously one of the problems with conversion of T4 to T3 is the presence of steroids in the body. Her body, under high amounts of stress was releasing large amounts of Cortisol, the body's natural steroid hormone. This was preventing the conversion of T4 to T3. I prescribed a low dose of Cytomel, which is a form of T3 and advised her to start lowering the stressors in her life she could control. The first stress lowering option I arranged for her was a free massage. This is a classic example of how the thyroid and adrenal glands depend on each other.

How to treat the thyroid gland:

If you are not able to utilize T3 because of any of the above reasons, the regular medications that are used that only contain T4 may not be for you. If that is the case, then take action and ask about Cytomel, which is T3, or better yet use Armour Thyroid. Armour Thyroid has **both** T3 and T4 in a specific ratio. The reason for this ratio found in Armour Thyroid is that T3 only hangs around for a few HOURS, while T4 hangs around for a few DAYS.

The two ingredients need to be at differing concentrations in the medicine to fulfill their rolls. The human body also has a ratio of these two hormones in the body. In addition, studies have shown that intestinal absorption of the combination is better than with T4 alone. Studies have also shown that just having T3 in a preparation improves the conversion of T4 to T3. If your body was the party, it's as if T3 is doing everything possible to make the party fun and to assure everything goes as planned. It just needed to be invited to the party. Just remember the rhyme "T3 is good for me!" Just tell your doctor the seemingly all knowing pharmaceutical rep that keeps telling him or her there is no need to order a T3, because the pharmaceutical company they work for has assured them that their medicine will normalize the TSH with only T4, is wrong.

Doses of Armour Thyroid can range anywhere from 30 mg/day to 240 mg/day. Just tell your doctor to give up the ghost, stop twitching, and start using the Armour Thyroid. It just makes good sense any way you slice it. In the past the only issue with Armour Thyroid was finding a manufacturer that would guarantee medications that actually gave you the doses they print on the label. However, manufacturers of Synthroid have done such a bang up job of squeezing out the competition, that there are only a handful of Armour Thyroid manufacturers left. The variability in quality has diminished and it is not an issue any longer. The kind of information I am writing is making its rounds so more manufacturers are putting out higher quality Armour Thyroid in the hopes of capturing more business.

> **Figure 16: Drugs that may affect your thyroid or your thyroid medication**
>
> Drugs that reduce thyroid hormone production:
> - Lithium
> - Iodine containing medications
> - Amiodarone (Cordarone)
>
> Drugs that reduce thyroid hormone absorption: (not good when it already has that problem!)
> - Sucralfate (Carafate)
> - Ferrous Sulfate (Slow Fe)
> - Cholestyramine (Questram)
> - Colestipol (Colestid)
> - Aluminum containing antacids
> - Calcium products
>
> Drugs that increase metabolism of Thyroxine: (This means less T4 is available for use once in the blood)
> - Rifampin (Rifadin)
> - Phenobarbital
> - Carbamazepine (Tegretol)
> - Warfarin (Coumadin)
> - Oral hypoglycemic agents
>
> Drugs that displace thyroid hormone from protein binding: (Thyroid medicine levels may get too high)
> - Furosemide (Lasix)
> - Mefenamic Acid (Ponstel)
> - Salicylates (aspirin or aspirin like substances)

When a patient is already on a medication that comes only in the form of T4 and the doctor wants to change to Armour Thyroid, the transition needs to be done with care, the same as when dealing with all medications that will be discontinued. The way to taper off of T4 is to increase the Armour Thyroid by 15 mg every 7 days, as you decrease the amount of the medication that only contains T4 by 25 mg. This is done every 7th day until the T4 dosage has reached zero. If, as an example, the dose of T4 was 100mcg, at the end of the fourth week the dose of T4 would be zero and the dose of the Armour Thyroid would be 60mg/day. This is the time when the doctor needs to continue titrating upwards every 10 days until the appropriate dose is reached. For the 100 mcg of T4 the equivalent dose of Armour Thyroid is 60 mg. After 30 days, the patient's labs need to be re-evaluated and the patient needs to be examined. The rule of thumb for simply titrating Armour Thyroid upwards is to change it every 10 days, checking the patient's vitals and overall medical examination.

The goal to starting thyroid medication therapy is to start low and titrate up. If you have a cortisol deficiency it is even more important to start low and titrate up slowly. Keep this in mind, testing for cortisol levels is part of the treatment for treating a hypothyroid patient. This is because if there is a cortisol deficiency it may cause the conversion of T4 to T3 to occur at a very fast rate, leading to a hyperthyroid condition. Under normal conditions the usual starting dose is 30 mg/day and can end up somewhere between 60-120 mg/day. Based on labs and how you are feeling, up to 240 mg/day may be required, checking back every 3-6 months for a physical and lab level check. I know this is confusing. I just want you to know the basics so you can light a fire under your doctors' buttocks and let him or her figure this entire scenario out. Weight management programs that have a doctor on staff that is able to see the patients every other week will always be the better choice when looking at weight management programs.

POW: *ABSOLUTELY, POSITEVLY NEVER LET A DOCTOR TREAT YOUR THYROID WITHOUT EVALUATING ALL THREE OF THE FOLLOWING LABS (AT A MINIMUM): T3, T4, AND A TSH.*

CHAPTER 8

Ever been told you were Anemic?

Anemia can be as confusing as it is simple all at the same time. Iron deficiency anemia is the most common nutritional deficiency worldwide! Think it is just a coincidence that obesity is so prevalent as well? Iron deficiency anemia is more common because in many cases it can be associated with your food intake as opposed to what you are able or unable to produce in the body, like glands and the production of hormones. Normally, men and women (women that are not menstruating) lose around 1mg per day of iron. Women on their period lose 0.6-2.5% more than that average per day. A person can be deficient in their iron stores and feel the symptoms associated with low iron without actually having a lab level that is out of the normal range. This is because the range provided in a lab panel is just that, a range or average across a large spectrum of values measured. This is the reason medical schools teach students to treat both the lab value as well as the patient. One person may have a "low normal" value and feel just fine. The next person through the door with the same value may have relatively severe symptoms.

There are two ways to measure iron we will discuss. One is the iron in your blood that is functional and referred to as your total iron. This form of iron is able to exert specific metabolic effects. The second form of iron that is measured is a value of the amount of stored iron in our bodies and is called ferritin. Both forms can be found in what is called an anemia profile. Once these iron stores are gone, a person is then classified as "iron deficient". Iron is directly involved in the production of hemoglobin. Hemoglobin attached to red blood cells is what carries oxygen away from the lungs to nourish the rest of the body. If anemia is left untreated, the hemoglobin concentrations in the body begin to fall. As you will read in the next paragraph, oxygen delivery plays a critical role in the burning of fat.

Figure 17: Factors that may lead to acquiring or becoming more susceptible to the anemic condition:

- Family and Ethnic History of having Anemia
- Drug and Toxic exposures to include: chloramphenicol, methyldopa, quinidine, and benzene
- Blood loss: gastrointestinal, urinary blood loss, frequent donation of blood: more than 2 units per year in women and 3 units per year in men (phlebotomy)
- Dietary: low intake of vitamins A, C, and B12, folic acid, thiamine, and pyridoxine which can lead to poor formation of hemoglobin. Excess intake of alcohol which can lead to riboflavin deficiency which ultimately leads to an inability of red blood cells to carry oxygen
- Specifically if someone is deficient in vitamin E this can affect the red blood cells membrane and it becomes fragile leading to hemolytic anemia (the cell membrane essentially breaks)
- Look at how rapid the onset of the anemia occurred: gradual onset leads to suspicion of bone marrow problems, where sudden onset leads one to suspect breakdown of blood cells or bleeding somewhere in the body suddenly
- A diet high in calcium can decrease the uptake of iron if both are taken at the same time

---

Figure 18: Other Risk Factors for Iron Deficiency Anemia in the U.S.
• Black Ethnicity
• Endurance Training
• Mexican Ethnicity living in the U.S.
• Low Socio-Economic Status
• Malabsorption (Celiac Disease)
• Adults that had experienced Child and Adolescent Obesity
• BMI > 85%
• Vegetarian Diet-40% of vegans 19-50 years old were Iron Deficient

My goal is for you to understand the enormous impact anemia can have on your ability to reduce your weight, not to learn how to self diagnose or treat the condition. Prior to beginning one of my weight management programs every patient undergoes a complete physical exam to include a **Resting Metabolic Rate**. If a clinic or commercial weight management center advertises how fast they can help you lose weight; yet they do not start the exam with a test of your metabolic rate, this should serve as your first sign you are in the wrong place. This test is a measurement of how much oxygen your body uses at rest. The next sentence is the major reason why it is so vital to make sure you are not anemic and if you are that it is treated correctly.

Every calorie you burn uses a **specific amount of oxygen** and measuring the resting metabolic rate is a great place to start in the investigation as to what is going on. **Let me repeat that**, every calorie you burn uses a specific amount of oxygen. Being anemic, even borderline anemic is unacceptable. Staying borderline anemic essentially means you will stay borderline fat. In other words if being borderline anemic is causing you to gain weight it is not borderline anymore is it. This is just another example of treating both the labs **and** the patient. It is also a testament to paying closer attention to lab levels that are "borderline low". There are simply not enough doctors out there who relate being anemic with gaining weight. As one can see it can have quite a bit to do with how a person handles a calorie.

Figure 19: Symptoms of Anemia
- Weakness, fatigue, or lack of stamina.
- Shortness of breath during exercise.
- Headache.
- Trouble concentrating.
- Irritability.
- Pale skin.
- Craving ice

Other signs may include:
- Rapid heartbeat.
- Brittle fingernails and toenails.
- Cracked lips.
- Smooth, sore tongue.
- Muscle pain during exercise.
- Trouble swallowing.

If the level of hemoglobin on and red blood cells in your blood are too low to carry all of the oxygen required by the body, then each person with anemia will consequently have a tough time reducing weight. In the type of anemia I am concerned with here, you can think of the anemic condition as being caused by two different scenarios. First, think of hemoglobin as a back pack your red blood cells carry. Each red blood cell carries four backpacks. The goal is to put an oxygen molecule into each of those four backpacks (hemoglobin is the back pack) as the red blood cells pass through the oxygen rich lungs. The second way to think about the cause of anemia is that there just are not enough individual red blood cells to carry those four backpacks. In other words, somewhere red blood cells are being destroyed or not being made.

If the resting metabolic rate comes out low, it does not tell the doctor what is specifically wrong, but at least the doctor knows that you need a complete workup. That includes what the problem might be with holding onto or having enough oxygen to burn fat efficiently and then ordering an anemia profile as a good first step. From the more rare forms of anemia such as Pernicious Anemia (not able to pull nutrients out of the food you eat) to the formerly discussed iron deficient and hemolytic anemia (red blood cells are fragile and break easily), you should be able to expect that your doctor understands how to diagnose anemia and is willing to treat the condition with an eye on your ability to burn fat.

Figure 20: Two Main Causes for Anemia

One: There is a decrease in production of red blood cells:

- Deficiency of nutrients and enzymes in the blood that allow production of red blood cells and hemoglobin in the blood.
- Bone marrow failure
- Kidney disease

Two: Increased red blood cell destruction or loss:

- Hemolytic or where hemoglobin is being released from red blood cells. It's like getting your backpack stolen at scout camp. It pisses you off but you really need to do something about it.
- Hemorrhage, or bleeding from somewhere in the body.

How to treat Anemia:

How does what we eat affect anemia? In many instances, when someone goes on a strict food program on their own, their intake of leafy green vegetables or lean meat may decrease. This is an important issue because iron is found in two forms in the foods we eat: heme and non-heme iron. Fish, chicken, and red meat have adequate stores of heme iron (easy to absorb). But non-heme iron (difficult to absorb) can also be found in animal meat and in plant stores. This kind of non-heme iron is absorbed to a much lesser degree. The good news is that combining the foods that have both types of heme iron can actually increase the absorption of both.

Vitamin C helps with the uptake of iron out of the intestines. If your diet contains foods that have iron which is difficult for your body to absorb, either take 500-1000mg of vitamin C per day or try to include foods high in vitamin C like strawberries, tomatoes, and bell peppers. These types of foods are what you should look for in any good food program. If I have a patient taking supplemental iron I will have them take both vitamin C and their Iron supplement at the same time to increase the uptake of the Iron. I know this all sounds a little confusing but that is your doctor's problem. He or she is supposed to be the one that went to medical school. This fact does not necessarily make him or her smarter. It just means they should be able to understand how to accomplish what I explain because this is their field of study. Your field of study may have been engineering. Asking your doctor the stress bearing joints of a bridge would be useless. It will be your job to remind your doctor you have anemia and to look for any of the possible reasons why this condition could be making it hard for you to lose weight.

This book is **written for the patient** so they can march to their doctor's office and expect some help in this process of replenishing the oxygen to their red blood cells, if anemia is suspected. As a weight management physician I offer injections of B12 (Cyanocobalamine), as well as a combination injection that has Methionine, Inositol, and Choline (MIC). The MIC injection increases sensitivity to insulin. I also offer multi-vitamins and sublingual B12 (2500-5000 mcg) combined with Folic Acid (800 mg) to my patients that are extremely bio-available. Taking B12 in any form other than as an injection or sublingual is close to useless. The simple fact is that the liver will breakdown the B12 when it is swallowed as a pill, called the "First Pass Effect". The amount you will receive in your blood will be lower than the amount taken, so just ask your doctor about this first pass effect. Glycine is an important supplement to take for the anemic person with low hemoglobin. It is involved in the **synthesis** of hemoglobin. Glycine is simply an amino acid, a building block of proteins involved in the synthesis of hemoglobin. With hemoglobin being the backpack that red blood cells use to put oxygen in as they flow through the lungs. Glycine helps your body build a brand name backpack. Research has indicated that Glycine in the dose range of 200 mg/Kg (of body weight)/day were the most effective at rendering the uptake and bio-availability of iron to adequate levels. Understand though that taking Glycine is not going to cure your anemia it is not that simple, medicine is never that simple. You may end up taking supplements for the rest of your life.

> **Figure 21: Tests that are ordered for diagnosing anemia:**
> - *CBC
> - *Serum Ferritin
> - Total Iron Binding Capacity
> - RDW
> - *Serum Iron Level
>
> *Most Important to be ordered

There are different methods to treat anemia. That is not the issue for you as the patient, the issue for you is being able to understand that weight management medicine is the answer, and anemia is just one of the possible issues at play preventing you from reducing weight. If you have a history of being borderline anemic, or your mother or father needed to take iron supplements an "Anemia Profile" should be included on the lab slip your doctor hands you.

Pernicious Anemia is a bit more serious and involves antibodies your body produces that prevents you from being able to absorb B12 out of your intestines. A couple of other reasons why you may not be able to get enough B12 are from alcoholism, *Helicobacter pylori* infection (the bacteria that causes ulcers), decreased absorption due to Crohns disease, and dietary (as in the case of strict vegetarians).

There are also medications that may cause B12 deficiency, like Metformin, Omeprazole, and Cholestyramine. Do not misunderstand the link between any of these medications and B12, because not everyone has this problem when they take these medications. On the contrary, I prefer my diabetic patients to be on Metformin because of its ability to make the body more sensitive to insulin and the medicines ability to cut down on sugar production in the liver. The main purpose for including this paragraph is to remind the reader to be aware that if there is a problem with availability of B12, medications need to be examined. B12 and folate are closely linked and both need to be checked if you hear the words "Macrocytic Anemia".

A summary of pernicious anemia: the problem with pernicious anemia will be that you will not be able to extract the necessary nutrients from the food you eat and transport them out of the gut to be used by your body to create appropriate B12 stores. You will need to have the B12 administered by a sublingual route; in other words, it gets absorbed through the mucosa of your jaw or by an intra-muscular injection. When given through these routes, more of the B12 ends up in your blood stream. This will avoid the "First Pass Effect" mentioned before which is where the liver breaks down the pills you swallow and leaves a smaller amount available for your body.

As a side note, if you are diagnosed with being anemic it is always a good idea to screen for possible cancers of the intestines. The risk of malignancy for those patients 65 years and older was 9 percent! As to whether you should undergo an endoscopy or colonoscopy (allows doctors to visualize both the upper and lower intestines) is a matter of symptoms, age, and a subject to discuss with your doctor. For those that are 50 years old, are anemic by way of their labs but lack any other symptoms, a colonoscopy is indicated.

Iron Sulfate of 300 mg contains 60 mg of elemental iron, where as 325 mg of iron Gluconate provides only 36 mg of elemental iron. It should also be noted that there is an increase in absorption with a more acidic environment. As mentioned above, it is best to administer iron therapy with vitamin C and avoid using antacids, proton pump inhibitors, and H2 blockers at the same time or within 2 hours of taking the iron. This is because these make the stomach less acidic for that short period of time that you want to take your medicines for anemia. It's not going to hurt anyone to hold off on their antacids for a couple of hours while they take their iron.

I understand that a lot of medical terminology was thrown out at you in the above paragraphs. This is because anemia is a serious condition that needs attention for a number of reasons. All that you, as a patient, need to understand is that it may be involved in your inability to lose weight. At the very least, you can write down or copy some of the symptoms and the laboratory tests listed in the box above and give them to your doctor to help them understand that you are an *aware* and knowledgeable patient.

POW: *IF YOU ARE ANEMIC IT IS EASY TO GAIN WEIGHT AND NEARLY IMPOSSIBLE TO LOSE IT. IF YOU HAVE LAB LEVELS THAT ARE BORDERLINE YOU WILL LIKELY BE BORDERLINE OVERWEIGHT. AN ANEMIA PROFILE IS ONE OF THE BASIC, REQUIRED PANELS EVERY DOCTOR IN WEIGHT MANAGEMENT SHOULD ORDER.*

CHAPTER 9

Having irregular periods and hair growing in odd places?

If so you could have Polycystic Ovarian Syndrome (PCOS) which is an endocrine disorder; in other words, a problem with the release of hormones in the body that can affect many other normal functions of the body. PCOS is a disorder that affects <u>1 in 15 women</u>, primarily **women of reproductive age**, and is a leading cause of infertility. In terms of a medical perspective 1 in 15 is a large number of women. Many of my colleagues have told me they don't see this diagnosis made very often in their clinics<u>. I on the other hand am looking a bit harder for it and the diagnosis shows up quite often, being responsible for many of the reasons a woman may not be able to reduce her weight.</u> PCOS seems to run in families, so if any females on your mother or father's side had it; this increases your chance of acquiring the disorder.

Not all women with PCOS have cysts on their ovaries. So a negative ultrasound of the ovaries (one that does not show cysts) <u>does not</u> rule out the diagnosis. The bottom line here is that overweight women are prone to PCOS and to make sure that you have your doctor rule out the possibility of this disorder. This is even a greater issue if you perceive any of the symptoms listed in this section going on in your body. Let your physician worry about all of the medical details that is their job.

Figure 22: Criteria and Symptoms of PCOS

PCOS may be present if one of the following three criteria is met:
- Problems with ovulation
- Excess androgen activity (Total Testosterone will be elevated)
- Ovaries with multiple cysts (by gynecologic ultrasound) although cysts are not necessary to make the diagnosis (I know, that doesn't make sense . . . and it should be called poly testosterone syndrome, or poly problems with ovulation syndrome)
- Other endocrine disorders are ruled out

Common symptoms of PCOS:
- Irregular, few, or absent menstrual periods
- Infertility, generally resulting from chronic lack of ovulation
- Excessive and increased body hair, typically in a male pattern, legs, upper lip, chin, chest
- Hair loss appearing as thinning hair on top of the head
- Acne, oily skin
- Obesity (one in two women with PCOS are obese, especially in the mid-section)
- Depression
- High blood pressure

Brown discoloration of skin on back of neck, under arms, and groin

As is usual for most ailments on this earth the smoking status of the woman always needs to be taken into consideration. In general, the androgen levels (male hormones) in smoking women tend to be higher than their non-smoking counterparts. However, I would not suggest trying to treat PCOS, weight management, and smoking cessation at the same time. Even though it is true that androgen levels may be higher in the smoking woman, I would not advise trying to quit smoking and also concentrate on reducing weight. Regardless of how serious a condition or habit may be, if too many aspects of a person's life are taken away, the effort required to lose weight will most likely be too much to handle.

In most women with PCOS, the onset of menstruation begins at a normal age, but month to month their bleeding is unpredictable in onset, duration, and amount. Signs of male hormone excess usually are noticed around the age that menstruation starts. One theory I support is that this disorder occurs because the ovaries are stimulated to produce an overabundance of male hormones (androgens), particularly testosterone. Yes the ovaries also produce testosterone. Research has shown that insulin resistance plays a major role in PCOS. PCOS has many symptoms and each person may present differently.

Figure 23: Lab values helpful in making the diagnosis of PCOS
- Androstenedione, Total and Free Testosterone, and Dehydroepiandrosterone sulfate which all would be elevated (measuring to confirm elevations of both total and free testosterone is more sensitive)
- Elevated fasting insulin levels, because up to 70% of women with PCOS are diabetic. In fact, it is thought that the insulin resistance may be the cause of the PCOS and this insulin resistance is found in both normal weight and overweight women
- Chronic inflammation is also found to be higher in people with PCOS. Therefore, inflammatory indicators like sedimentation rates should be ordered

---

Like many of the other disorders in this book I have provided lists of labs you may need, I do not expect you to understand what the levels mean or how elevated or low they need to be to cause problems. All I expect is for you to highlight these levels and bring the book into the clinic and show your doctor what you fully expect him or her to measure. Keep in mind that we should not base any diagnosis on the results of just one lab or just one symptom. As you can tell, some of these disorders I have written about are not the easiest to diagnose and treat. You need to look for doctors that see the big picture and feel comfortable thinking outside the confines of the normal medical box. A doctor may start out with their mind set on one diagnosis and not be open to others that may almost mirror the symptoms and some of the labs of the actual diagnosis. When this "other" diagnosis is solely pursued, the actual problem goes untreated. Not only does the doctor have to take the time to figure this entire scenario out, he or she then needs to take the time and patience to explain to you what is going on in your body. The patient needs to know and be told that the weight gain or inability to get weight off is not their fault and explain what is wrong. This takes TIME, a lot more time than most doctors are accustomed to giving to one patient in one visit. Never doubt that you are worth this time. The doctor chose medicine, medicine is the cure for obesity and you deserve the cure.

A PCOS patient example:

A woman walked in for a consultation on reducing weight. She was 48 years old, and I notice she had a bit of acne. I asked her if she had any hair on her chest or around her nipples. She embarrassingly answered, "Yes." I then looked at her chart and noticed that she had one of her ovaries removed. I simply asked her why they had performed the surgery. She said her ovaries had cysts on them and that the one they removed was the most painful. The problem was that this was the full extent of her treatment. They did not address any of the other underlying symptoms of PCOS which ovarian cysts were only one! After running the appropriate laboratory panels I confirmed the diagnosis and began to treat Poly Cystic Ovarian Syndrome, which meant controlling her levels of testosterone, sugar, insulin, and staying on top of the hormone abnormalities that will surely creep in as she begins pre-menopause. Because I went further than just the "band-aid" approach of removing a painful ovary, we were able to start the journey of successful weight management.

How to treat PCOS:

Women with PCOS have a very difficult time getting pregnant. This is because they have a consistently high level of a hormone called luteinizing hormone (LH). LH is normally supposed to surge which causes progesterone to go up, which then causes the uterine lining to thicken as it prepares for ovulation and implantation of an egg. Because LH levels stay elevated throughout the cycle, the normal menstrual cycle with release of an egg is interrupted. Therefore, infertility is just another condition the female has to deal with.

This condition is not an easy one to diagnose. This is mainly because it can vary so much in severity and can mirror other disorders. This is why a lot of physicians early on when faced with a female who is not interested in getting pregnant, has irregular periods, and may even have all of the other symptoms of PCOS, will simply start them on the birth control pill. In the case of a thin patient the doctor may not even think to look into a possible diagnosis of PCOS. PCOS may even be over looked in the overweight female if the only presenting symptom is irregular menstruation. In my experience the norm is a reactive medical approach where the doctor does not even begin a search for a problem until the patient is obese, growing hair on her face and chest, has ample amounts of discoloration under her arms, and becomes diabetic. At this point a second year medical student could make the diagnosis . . . ugh. I really have grown tired of seeing this. I am not against using the birth control pill. The pill has some advantages that are listed in figure 22. I'm just against medical ignorance.

Figure 24: What is the purpose and expectations from initiation of the birth control pill?

- May regulate the menstrual cycle if tolerated
- Attempts to correct the hormone imbalances. But, as many women will attest, some women cannot tolerate the pill. If the woman can tolerate the pill, they can expect a lowering of the testosterone level
- Lowering the testosterone will help the acne and possibly the hair growth
- Lowers the risk of endometrial cancer, because this type of cancer is more common in women who do not ovulate
- In sexually active women, it may prevent an unplanned pregnancy
- May worsen the overweight condition (I know, I know it's a double edged sword to say the least)

Birth control pills may regulate the periods, but it does very little for the overweight condition. Birth control pills <u>may actually worsen the overweight condition</u>. Even though the irregular periods are taken care of with the pill, the sugar that is still left in the blood secondary to the insulin resistance is still an issue. The sugar that isn't stuck in your arteries is brought to the liver, converted to fat, and stored throughout the body. Therefore, the insulin resistance needs to be addressed: **this means the weight management needs to be addressed**. If the normal reactive approach to treatment continues and the weight management ignored, this overweight patient will eventually be a patient with PCOS and diabetes. <u>One study showed that 40% of women with PCOS had full blown diabetes by the age of 40!</u>

As I said before, the doctor gets rid of or puts a Band-Aid on the irregular periods but is not thinking out of the medical box at the bigger picture. The questions that needed to be asked were, "*What was causing the irregular periods?*"; "*Why are her hormones so unpredictable?*", and if the female is overweight "*Why is she so heavy?*"

A study conducted in 2000 showed a higher risk of coronary heart disease in women with PCOS.[2] This is because they found higher levels of the "bad cholesterol" (or LDL) and high blood pressure (think insulin resistance and high sugar could be involved??). They also found atherosclerotic plaques (basically blockages, or soon to become blockages in the blood vessels) on the interior walls of the arteries, showing that there was a definitive link between heart disease and having PCOS. Not only this, they found in women age 45 and older the plaques were thicker. Here it is again, an example of the importance of finding a doctor to treat you that looks at the whole person and the big picture OR YOU WILL GET SICKER!

Many physicians disagree on the best way to test for PCOS. Most will rule out other diseases first like Cushing's disease, Congenital Adrenal Hyperplasia (talk about the zebra causing the hoof beats?!), and increased prolactin production by the pituitary. Testing for all of the zebras is not a problem as long as you the patient are assured that the basic labs that will help diagnose PCOS are also ordered. At the very least a total and free testosterone level needs to be ordered (they will be elevated) as well as a total insulin level (which will be elevated as well).

When treating PCOS in conjunction with treating the obese condition, <u>increasing the sensitivity to insulin is an important goal</u>. Many physicians say insulin resistance is the root cause of PCOS. The first conservative measure is the starting of a low glycemic index diet (choosing the right kinds of carbohydrates) in which the <u>lowering of weight</u> will help to restore normal ovulation/ menstruation. The lower carbohydrate foods will also help lower the levels of insulin by lowering the requirements for insulin.

There is a newer treatment rarely employed referred to as ovarian drilling, which is performed laparoscopically. A laser fiber or electrosurgical needle is used to puncture the ovary 10-12 times. This treatment results in a dramatic lowering of male hormones (testosterone) within days. Studies have shown that up to 80% of women will benefit from such treatment. Many women who failed after trying insulin lowering therapy began to respond to these medications after this procedure.

When looking at which medications may be of use, Metformin is at the top of the list. This medicine alone will usually restore ovulation once the insulin resistance begins to resolve and insulin levels in the blood drop. This also aids in weight management because remember, insulin as the ultimate enemy, hinders weight reduction. Some other positive effects of Metformin are that it has been shown to reduce male pattern hair growth, acne, and corrects menstrual irregularities. But (yes there is always a but) remember that in addition to the above therapies, eating correctly and exercising are what I would call the trinity of weight management when these two are combined with adequate water intake.

Since hair growth is a sensitive issue, other treatments that focus on this include Eflornithine (Vaniqua). This is a cream that is applied to the areas that are growing the hair. This is usually applied to the face. Another two oral medications are flutamide and spironolactone. The latter is a diuretic, and is the most commonly used in the US for this type of hair growth in women.

An alternative, more natural approach to the treatment of PCOS in general is the use of D-Chiro-Inositol (DCI). This is not a drug but instead a nutrient that has been proven in two studies to positively affect insulin metabolism, decrease the production of male pattern hair growth, decrease blood pressure and triglyceride levels. This nutrient should be used at 1200mg once daily. Once these measures are begun, you will begin to feel better. This is the time to start a weight management program, as well as an adequate exercise regimen. It may be the first time in a long time you have been able to lose weight.

In summary staying healthy and fit is a never-ending battle. I have written about a few of the more prevalent disorders involved in the battle against obesity. There are others and I will no doubt feel the need to write about those as well. This is a start. I have started with the disorders I have found to be the main culprit in the vast majority of women and men I have treated. Take what I have written and begin to push towards a much needed paradigm shift in the medical field. The shift needs to be one that replaces the current REACTIVE APPROACH to medicine with a PROACTIVE APPROACH that fosters health instead of sickness. Reading this book and becoming your own best health advocate by taking your proactive plan to the doctor is just a small part. The goal is keeping the weight off for the rest of your life. Change is inevitable: change in our bodies, change in our environment. Resistance is futile! You, as a patient, need to be looking ahead at what you will do to keep the weight off once menopause or andropause (for the men) hits. The best you can do is learning how to make those changes as pleasant an experience as possible. No doctor no matter how knowledgeable regarding weight management can help you keep the weight off if you decide to go back to bad eating habits and decrease your exercise. There is no magic wand or pill you can take for life that will keep the weight off while you do whatever you want. It takes hard work and constant attention to get and keep the body and health you desire.

POW: FOR THIS DISORDER THE MOST IMPORTANT ISSUES ARE THE PHYSICAL SIGNS AND SYMPTOMS. READ THEM CAREFULLY AND SEE IF THEY CORRELATE WITH WHAT YOU SEE AND FEEL IN YOUR OWN BODY.

CHAPTER 10

Are our Children becoming Obese?

Ultimately, if we focus more attention on this group, it would have enormous effects on the obesity epidemic. This is because one of the most important aspects in the treatment of this group is including the parents' in the child's eating and exercise patterns. It is no coincidence that I ended the last section on PCOS, a disorder commonly discovered early in life. Parents are responsible for the welfare of their children until that child moves out and on with their lives. This not only includes the obvious necessities of life like providing a loving environment, food and shelter. This also includes being aware of what may be wrong medically when their child seems to be gaining weight.

It is imperative that the parents offer support and non-judgmental acceptance. This is important for proper psychological development which, if not dealt with appropriately, will spill over into adulthood negatively. No patient or doctor should want a child to remain overweight and be exposed to the cruel jokes, teasing, and low self-esteem. Many studies have shown that overweight/obese girls have extremely low self-esteem, trouble getting into college, and have a difficult time with social interactions.

As these kids grow into adults, they are more likely to remain overweight or obese and carry all of those associated disease risks with them. Studies have shown numbers as high as seventy percent of the children that are obese continue in that condition into adulthood! It is essential that pediatricians take control of these kids. I have had enough of hearing "they'll grow out of it" statements. Yes, it is true that they indeed may grow out of it. They will not grow out of it if they continue to increase their intake and gain weight along with their increase in height and stature. The rule of thumb that "They will grow out of it" stems from the fact that if parents can keep the child the same weight as they grow, it is equivalent to losing five pounds per inch of height attainment! The question is how long and at what age of very little or no growth does the pediatrician wait to address the obesity issue.

Obese children experience many health problems at increasingly early ages. Pain in the joints and back and global inflammation is being seen in this age group at levels higher than ever before. Type II Diabetes Mellitus is now being diagnosed in the young. This disorder was previously referred to as Adult Onset Diabetes Mellitus. This is because it was adults that carried extra weight into middle age that ended up with Diabetes. It is difficult to diagnose a 16 year old with *Adult Onset Diabetes*. Just like an adult, a child's weight gain is predictive of the disease processes they will have to deal with. It is tough to get a child outdoors playing when they are in pain.

The simple fact that the child is obese could mean there is an underlying disorder with their hormones or a host of other problems. The typical pediatric work-up will not apply to these obese kids. It is vital to look closely at the family history of medical disorders. Disorders that are rare can be addressed such as Prader-Willi and Lawrence-Moon-Biedel, but the more common disorders occur, well, more commonly. Many of the disorders covered in this book may occur in children as well as adults, and should not be ignored.

Pediatricians will run into a number of problems while trying to treat kids. Some of these are as simple as time constraints when counseling the child and the parents. It is very difficult to keep a child's attention. When you are talking about taking away their french fries, it is even tougher. There are very few medically supervised pediatric weight management programs available that do not require a large output of upfront money by the doctor. However, just getting to a point where nutrition is better understood by the parents is a huge step forward.

Parental involvement is vital! However, the problem with parental involvement is that it is very hard to achieve. If both parents work, the intervention of the parents is more difficult. The same is true for single parents. In this situation, the parent is tired and may not feel like cooking; therefore, the child may consume a large quantity of fast food. Single parents also have a difficult time scheduling a regular exercise program or involving the child in a sport. A sport requires the parent to a commitment of transport, time, and support. It may come easy to some but there are plenty that seem to find every reason in the world why they just cannot find the time to get their kids involved.

When doctors attempt to rely on the children to keep track of their intake and exercise, doctors find the same problems as with adults. The kid's overestimate their time spent exercising and underestimate the amount they are eating. It is very difficult to treat a patient when you have information that is not reliable.

When doctors treat obese children, they have to be especially aware of how low to go on the calorie count. If too low, there is a risk of slowing growth. The better way is to make sure the child does not eat the wrong type of foods, like high (sugar) glycemic index foods. If a child is hitting a growth spurt, then nutrient intake may need to be increased or the child taken off of the program. This is because during these times of growth, if the child is exposed to decreased macro- and micro-nutrient intakes, linear growth can slow down.

In our youth we will find similar problems as with adults: there is a shortage of physical activity. This is made worse with all of the video games and internet activity at their fingertips that are difficult for the parents to control. The recommendations for exercise are the same as adults, with thirty minutes of activity at least four days per week. It is tough these days to simply tell our children to go outside and find something to do with criminal activity so prevalent. It is not like it used to be in the seventy and eighties when our parents could say, "Get out of the house. Be back before the street lights come on." Keeping our children active and busy requires effort on the part of the parent. Parents should encourage and assist kids in participating in sports, working out at the gym, or just "hanging out" with friends outside and near the house. There is a unique way I have learned to help those of us with children take a more active role in the amount of food your child eats. When serving food to your children place small, but healthy portions of the different foods involved in a meal on the child's plate. When the child is done eating that smaller portion ask the child if they would like another serving or are they satisfied enough to take part in a favorite activity. If the child is truly satisfied they will usually opt for taking part in that favorite activity. If they do ask for another serving give it to them. As this is repeated you will slowly gain a better understanding of how many calories the child is accustomed to taking in at each meal. You will then be able to adjust this intake as you are tracking their growth pattern and weight changes.

If you are worried that your child will start smoking to replace eating, there is one strong deterrent for those children who are conscious of their appearance. People who smoke increase the amount of fat that is deposited on their chest and abdominal region. This fact may be a more effective deterrent than the risks of cardiovascular diseases and cancer. But do not let the doctor sit on the weight gain and do nothing. Make sure that there is nothing wrong hormonally or otherwise with your child, especially if there is anything in your family history that may explain the weight gain. Do not try to determine on your own if it is significant or not, just tell your doctor everything. It is the doctors' job to determine if there are hormone problems or some other type of medical issue at play. It is your job to make sure the doctor is aware that you are an educated parent and that your child has some of the same symptoms as one of the disorders in this book and you want an appropriate work-up started. With the alarming increase in the number of kids being diagnosed with type II diabetes a lot of informational web sites have emerged. Get out there and do your due diligence. If not for yourself then do it for your children.

> *POW: WITH CHILDREN IT IS NOT NECESSARY TO PUT THEM ON A DIET. REMEMBER THAT FOR EVERY INCH THEY GROW, IT IS EQUIVALENT TO LOSING 5 POUNDS. THIS IS TRUE AS LONG AS THE ACTUAL WEIGHT DOES NOT CHANGE.*

CHAPTER 11

Is it all in My Head or Society's Fault?

This next section will deal with the issues most would classify under the psychological. Issues that physicians need to take the time to help their patients get through. It is a step that is just as important as figuring out medically why their patient is overweight or obese. This is when the choice needs to be made as to whether the doctor is willing to take the time to treat these psychological issues on their own instead of referring them to a specialist. If the physician is not willing to take this time then weight gain again is not the patients fault. It is the fault of the providers who are responsible for treating all of the health issues related to the obese condition. The health problems I have written about previously are just as important as the psychological components in this section. Prior to Nestle' acquiring Novartis Medical Nutrition, in 2002 Novartis trained me in the basics of nutritional science and patient care during the Active Weight Management Phase. This training established the groundwork upon which many of the topics I discuss in the following pages were built.

Treating these issues is where the rubber meets the road, where medicine meets weight reduction. It's one thing to order some labs, make a diagnosis, and treat it with a prescription or over the counter supplement. It is quite another to do this and then take the time to address those psychological problems that will without a doubt wreak havoc on any weight management program whether the correct diagnosis was correct or not. These issues and the discussion of them are what can take the most time in the long run of any clinic visit. I plan on discussing the issues I have dealt with the most and what I have found to work the best at resolving them. Some are a combination of both physical (for instance feeling hungry when you are low on nutrients) and psychiatric (feeling hungry when you smell the next door neighbor grilling steaks). Or the difference in feeling depressed because you are overweight, and feeling depressed because you are chemically low on serotonin in your brain. So let's go.

Night Eating Syndrome:

An interesting point associated with hunger I want to cover is something called Night Eating Syndrome (NES). Normally the sleeping patterns of humans are set such that night time food intake does not occur. The synchronization of these rhythms is set by a central pacemaker in the middle of our brain. In some of us there seems to be a breakdown of the patterns of eating and sleeping. There are links between stress and the onset of NES, and elevated levels of cortisol. This may precipitate awakenings and the onset of eating during these times, sort of a form of self-soothing stress management. This in turn may help lead to the overweight/obese condition. There are two medicines that have shown some promise in this area. One is Wellbutrin at 150 mg before bedtime, and Sertraline (Zoloft) starting at 25mg prior to bedtime and slowly increasing the dose as needed. This should probably be under the "Disorders that go unnoticed" section, but I put it here because it needs to be under the section of eating the wrong foods at the wrong time; and the amount of exercise it takes to burn calories. This syndrome will pop up again when we talk about healthy speeds of weight management.

> *POW: ABOVE ALL ELSE (ASIDE FROM HORMONE DISORDERS) EXERCISE WILL PROVIDE THE MOST RESTFUL SLEEP.*

Hunger:

The biggest mistake people have been making for years is taking appetite suppressants and not eating. It is not that I don't prescribe these medicines, because I do. The worse favor a doctor can do is to practice weight management medicine by handing out appetite suppressants and simply telling their patients to eat less and exercise more. There is a WORLD of information that each person needs to be given and have explained to help them keep the weight off once they are done losing it. This would be impossible at just one visit to your primary care doctor. This information needs to be presented over a period of time. It is too late once the patient has lost the weight and headed into maintenance. In the end it is going to come down to how the patient lost the weight and are they prepared physically and mentally to keep it off.

I am not saying that a self motivated person would not lose weight if they were simply put on an appetite suppressant, given a "Diabetic Food Program", and told to drink water and exercise because they just might. The problem with these types of programs is that the patients' burn up muscle, lower their metabolic rate and gain all of their weight back plus some if everything is not done right. To further explain this scenario let's do it by way of example. Let's say you have a metabolism that burns 1100 calories per day. You have been eating 2000 calories each day and gaining weight in the process. You go to your doctor or worse yet you go thru the internet and get some appetite suppressants. You do what you assume you are supposed to do by cutting way back on your eating. Most people end up eating less than 1000 calories per day, or if they are eating more than this it is usually non-nutritious. This amount of food and usually the types of food only serve to burn up muscle. I am not saying that you would not burn up fat, you would. But you would also be burning up muscle; thereby making it nearly impossible to keep the weight off once the goal weight is achieved. Since this person is burning up muscle, and muscle weighs more than fat it tends to look good on the scale. Since muscle represents 30-40% of the metabolic rate they get a big surprise when they try to go back to eating what they used to eat when they were at a normal weight. Because they have burned so much muscle their metabolic rate can now only burn 700-800 calories. Therefore even at a calorie count of only 1000 calories weight gain begins.

When the body is low on protein because a diet is non-nutritious, it simply breaks down lean tissue to get the protein it needs. During weight management all looks well on the scale because when you are dealing with the *same volume of tissue* muscle weighs more than fat. Let me put it another way, if we take as an example two abdomens that are the exact same size. Then we assume one of these abdomens has a preponderance of fat, while the other fills the same volume of abdomen with muscle. If everything aside from the abdomens was the same and we were to weigh these two individuals the person with the muscular abdomen will weigh more! Muscle is also more metabolically active than fat. Whatever percent of muscle the person burned while dieting will be the percent drop in their metabolic rate. When all is said and done this drop in metabolism will result in weight gain. This is when you hear the same old song, "I gained all of my weight back plus 10 pounds". Why does weight gain occur if the person is eating the same amount of calories they used to eat when they were at their previous weight prior to gaining the weight? It is because when they were eating let us just say, 1200 calories they had enough lean muscle to burn this caloric intake. Unfortunately they are now left with less muscle mass than they previously had because their intake was too low and their body burned muscle to make up the difference. Now when you hear people say "I've done so many crazy diets that I know I have messed up my metabolism" you can explain just how true that is.

Why does insulin go up when you are eating less? Most people, if they know anything about insulin, know that it goes up when we eat. This rise in insulin occurs because your body goes into a self preservation mode. When your intake is too low, the physiologic mechanism in place to assure that your brain and muscles get the appropriate molecule to burn for energy kicks in. It is our liver that begins making this molecule. What is this wonderful molecule that triggers an insulin response, it is sugar. Yes, when your intake drops to a critical level your body is able to make sugar whether you are eating it or not. As was explained previously insulin is released in response to any load of sugar that gets deposited in the blood. Whether that sugar is dumped into the blood by the liver or by what we eat, the end result is the same, a rise in insulin levels. Go back to the diabetes section to read how difficult insulin can make weight management.

So when I prescribe appetite suppressants of any kind I make a very serious deal with the patient. The deal is that no matter how they feel they will eat what is on their food program. The appetite suppressant is there simply to make the job a little easier. Now we should discuss the different types of hunger and where they come from. Appetite suppressants are covered in more detail further on in the book.

What is the physiology and psychology of hunger?

Well there are a number of reasons a person can feel satisfied with a meal. One is called the vagal stretch. This is a nerve wrapped around the stomach. When it gets stretched it sends a signal to your brain that you are full. Another way we feel full is by way of a hormone referred to as Leptin. This is a hormone that will send a signal to the brain that you have eaten enough. This hormone is released after around 20 minutes, so if you take your time eating Leptin will do its' job. Of course you may be Leptin resistant but that is a different story. The type of hunger most relevant to discuss and more difficult to understand, is the type that is stimulated by an actual lack of needed nutrients. In this type of hunger either macro-nutrients or micro-nutrient levels are low, and the body is trying to tell you it is time to eat. Sometimes you may even feel cravings for certain foods. This is because the body has learned over the years which types of foods contain the nutrients your body requires.

The amazing part of all of this is that the reason it is so hard to tell if you are truly hungry or not is because there is only one hunger center. If you get a smell of steak, that hunger signal goes to the same place as the hunger signal from the stomach that is telling you, you really are hungry because you lack nutrients. So that smell of steak or seeing that steak cooking will send a surge of insulin into your blood and from the above reading you now know that insulin makes you hungry! They take different paths to get to that hunger center. One way is through the outside part of the mid-brain and the other is through the inside area. The trick has always been to try and find a drug that blocked both sides, but didn't harm us in any way.

We have to beware of eating in response to how food may make us feel. <u>Sweets actually do increase certain hormones in the brain that make us feel less depressed</u>. Sweets can increase the levels of serotonin, the same brain chemical raised when people take Prozac as well as many other anti-depressants. Research has also shown that having very harsh cravings that are difficult to control may be because of a low level of dopamine. Wellbutrin is a medicine that can help to raise the levels of dopamine. Research has found that the people most susceptible to addictions to drugs in general are the ones with measured low levels of dopamine. The important part to remember is that eating in response to these signals really can be an addiction that is treatable. People throw around the phrase that "I am addicted to eating'. Most people do not understand that they indeed are addicted to food in a very biologically specific way. This may lead a person to an over indulgence in the food that fulfills the craving signal coming from the brain.

When you are on a low calorie program your body senses that there is a low supply of food, or that you must be in the midst of a famine. This is just good old evolution at work. Therefore when you cheat and eat something the hunger will REALLY kick in. The body is trying to tell you to eat as much as you can since you have obviously found this new food source in the midst of this famine it thinks you are in. Carbohydrates are the worse to cheat with because most of the types we tend to cheat with are simple carbohydrates that raise our blood sugar and subsequent insulin levels.

The effect of sugar on a weight management program is bewildering and at times extremely frustrating. When we eat sugars they can be converted to their storage form of glycogen and stored in our muscles and liver. When this glycogen is deposited in your muscles water will follow. This is why we can feel a bit bloated when we eat more than we should. Then what happens is the next time you decide to really behave and exercise hard, instead of burning lots of fat like you are thinking your body is doing, it is burning that stored sugar or "glycogen" and leaving the fat alone. This makes sense also, because the preferred energy for muscle is glycogen and when you are exercising you are obviously using those muscles. Why would those muscles use a less efficient form of energy such as fat when that sugar has been made so readily available by your cheating? When you weigh yourself after all of your hard work you will not have lost anything. This can really send some people into a tail spin. Especially when I tell them they did great this week, but because of the previous weeks cheating, they simply need to repeat that hard work again. As long as there is no cheating, instead of simply burning that glycogen and water they will actually force their body into burning fat. When they come to the office how would I even know what their body was burning for energy? Because I can measure body fat percent, as well as total body water, their weight and compare these values to the previous week.

The way to deal with cheating is to be honest with yourself and admit that you overate and what it was that you ate. If it was carbohydrate in nature the best way to battle the delay in burning fat is to do a resistance training circuit at your fitness center. One thing you NEVER do is starve yourself for the next two days after you cheat. That is one of the worst things you can do. You need to bite the bullet, go back to your food program the way it was written by your doctor, drink water and exercise a bit more the days following the cheating. Starving yourself does nothing but slow down your metabolism even further. Remember exercise will <u>always </u>be the key.

One thing to understand about hunger is that when you are paying attention to your intake and have been doing well, this may be when the fiercest hunger strikes. In these situations hunger will be accompanied with feeling fatigued and having cravings. This will not make any sense if you stop and evaluate what you have been doing. If you have been eating correctly, drinking your water, and exercising regularly you will know intuitively you should not be feeling this way. Stop and think about the best way for the body to prevent fat burning? Because even though fat may be unhealthy, evolutionarily fat is supposed to be what gets us through famine and those harsh winter months. So in spite of how much we would enjoy our body to willingly rid itself of fat, the answer during those times when we are about to start a serious fat burning phase will always be to make you hungry. Evolutionarily we have not evolved past the point where our bodies react to excess fat by willingly burning it for energy. Our bodies still store fat so we can make it through the winter, as if we were still in the pre-historic era. In actuality this is the week where you stand to lose the most weight. I tell my patients to try their best to push through this time and the pay off can be big. If they can continue to drink their water and stay within their calorie count they will lose a lot of weight. This is when trust comes into place and the patient just needs to believe that the weight management program they are on is healthy and their hard work will pay off.

It has also proven helpful to eat foods served hot. This is secondary to the fact that you will usually eat them more slowly and take smaller bites. I want you to take at least twenty minutes to finish a meal. This is around the minimal time it takes for the satiety signs (feeling satisfied) to reach your brain. While we are talking about hot food try hot chocolate (in moderation) or hot tea, The Journal of Agricultural and Food Chemistry has reported that these types of drinks contain more anti-oxidants than red wine. You should be able to find both of them listed on a weight management program. You would be hard pressed to find a wine that is geared for those looking to lose weight, regardless of how heart healthy wine may be. I am not saying you should never drink wine. I am saying there are better alternatives when you are trying to lose weight. Once you are in maintenance, wine can then be drunk in moderation (no pun intended).

POW: YOU WILL NEVER BE ABLE TO BE COMPLETELY DEVOID OF HUNGER DURING WEIGHT REDUCTION, ESPECIALLY IN THE FIRST 2 WEEKS. ACTUALLY IT IS AN IMPORTANT SENSATION THAT NEEDS TO BE DEALT WITH REASONABLY.

More hunger tips:

I would like to write about some tricks to keep you from feeling hungry or how to get to a satisfied state faster. Most of these tips I already knew and have used for years, but we can thank the media (for once) for a few that I thought were very interesting. If you want to add some fruit to your shake use blueberries they are one of the most fiber filled low glycemic index fruits on my food list with around 8 grams of fiber per cupful. It may be hard to believe but eating in a place where there is dim lighting will usually result in eating more. So eat in well lit places.

Remember fiber and that there are two types: water soluble, and water insoluble. To feel fuller you would want to eat more <u>water soluble fiber</u>: flax seed, apples, carrots, psyllium husk, and oat bran. To help get rid of constipation you want the <u>water insoluble fiber</u>: green beans, in general dark green leafy vegetables, whole wheat products. The water insoluble fiber will keep more water inside your GI tract promoting regular bowel movements. This movement of food through your intestines is a pretty important fact. It helps to prevent colon cancer. We really do not want stool sitting in our colon for days.

Since sight and smell also signals hunger (maybe not so much after discussing bowel movements . . .) try to not take big whiffs of warm brownies, and try not to look at them either. Ok, if those last few sentences fail to make you lose your appetite nothing will. Both sight and smell will trigger an insulin release and I've wrote above how dangerous insulin is to weight management and maintenance. If you are right handed, try eating with your left hand. It will probably guarantee you take at least 20 minutes to finish that meal. To also help you reach that 20 minutes try listening to soft, mellow music. You'll find yourself thinking about the day and pondering and giving that food time to digest. After every bite set the fork down and have a sip of water. If you are sitting next to someone try to talk a little in between each bite also. If you usually have a cocktail with your meals and really don't care for the harder liquors, wine has been shown to trigger the eating of larger portions more so than beer. But go for the light beer please.

Corn has too much natural sugar to be on my programs. But popcorn is all right once in a while at the movies, but watch the sodium and do not put butter on it! POP Secret has 100 calorie packs. I've mentioned this before, but it's worth another mention regarding night time hunger. Save a high protein medical shake for later on in the evening and add some frozen low GI fruit to it along with ice and water to bulk it up. When you are in maintenance and you are a pasta lover, white pasta will have your blood sugar dropping and you'll be hungry again quickly. Why, because of the insulin surge. Instead go for wheat pasta and the feeling of satisfaction will last MUCH longer, and it is flat out healthier for you.

Prior to dinner there are two things I would like for you to consider. Number one is having a 100 calorie medical shake 30 minutes before dinner. The other is to have a 100-150 calorie salad before dinner. Both will help you eat around 12-15% fewer calories of the dinner. Over the last few years patients have divulged that if they eat the same amount of fish or lean meat/turkey/chicken, they feel fuller with the fish. Fish has a lot of protein and of protein, carbohydrates, and fats it is the protein that will make you feel the most satisfied. Sleeping is very important, sleep deprived individuals have lower Leptin levels and higher hormones that produce hunger; try to get in 7-8 hours per night if possible. If eating out and you begin to feel satisfied have the waiter remove whatever you have not finished so you do not continue to pick at the food. Room temperature is also an issue believe it or not. When you are in a colder environment you will tend to eat more, so keep the thermostat in your house a little warmer as mealtimes approach.

Snacking:

Let's just look at how many calories can stack up when even small amounts of ingested calories go unanswered with exercise. Looking at 25 calories, (this may be the time to whip out the calculator) which are say 6 jelly beans, or an extra bite or two in a given meal. In order to perform this calculation you will need one additional piece of information. It requires 3500 calories to make one pound of fatty tissue. If you multiply those 25 calories of jelly beans by the 365 days in a year you get 9125 calories you have eaten in a year *and not burned off.* You then divide the 9125 calories by the 3500 calories (which is equivalent to one pound of fat) and you end up with an <u>extra 2.5 pounds of fatty tissue per year</u>. The reason this is so alarming is because it sort of sneaks up on you over time.

You can't see it daily because it is really only ounces that you are gaining daily. Then after 4 years have passed you have gained 10 pounds. It gets really scary when you look at the ten year mark and you have actually gained 25 pounds from eating 6 jelly beans per day!

Keep in mind that in the following scenario the person is **only over eating by 25 calories per day.** The amount usually over eaten in any given day on average is much more than this. Remember the name of this book is **when** weight gain is not your fault. There are patients that simply overeat and do not exercise enough to burn off those calories. They need to be taught about nutrition and exercise and pushed in the right direction weekly. That is no easy task for doctor's that have spent their entire career simply treating the effects of obesity like diabetes and high blood pressure, instead of treating the obesity as the fulcrum of treatment. This requires a balancing act of the medicines their patient is on with what they need to be eating, how much they need to exercise and how much water to drink. Then adjusting one side or the other so everything stays in balance and the patient continues to feel good and loses weight.

When you snack it is vital to at least take note of what it is you are snacking on. If they are primarily carbohydrates then there is a way to deal with this situation. Remember the way NOT to deal with an episode of snacking is by not eating the next day. This will only serve to lower your metabolism even further. Always know that in order to burn anything in your body, for any chemical reaction to take place water and nutrients are needed. In other words you need to eat but if you play, you will pay.

The way you handle snacking especially if it was with carbohydrates is with exercise. Not just any exercise. You need to find a circuit where you work your entire body using high repetitions and 2-3 sets. To be a bit more specific on this you need to separate out two days of the next week where you plan on doing a circuit of resistance training. You need to use low weight and high repetitions of around 12-15. Your muscles need to be "feeling the burn" by the last couple of repetitions or the weight you are using is too light.

This will burn off the glycogen stored in your muscles. You should also be doing your cardiovascular walking on the other days of the week. If you do the circuit twice and keep up with your walking you will not gain any weight. The hard part is that you will not lose either, and will have to wait till the next week to see the weight come off again. If you do not belong to a fitness center then simply perform the exercises I have written later in the book with the Bosu, Swiss ball, and a pair of light dumbbells at a fast pace. It is critical to have a complete history and physical exam and be cleared for exercise by your primary care provider.

I never have my patients cut out everything when they start my program, or get extremely strict with their intake. If too much is excluded from a person's life all at once it is usually a psychological shock to the system and they end up having a very hard time getting started on a smooth track to reducing weight. If they love having a diet soda with their dinner then I will tell them to continue. If they have coffee in the morning I will not have them discontinue this. The last thing they need is a carbohydrate withdrawal headache on top of a caffeine withdrawal headache; they'll think they're having a stroke or something. It's important to understand that when a person stops drinking enough water and their exercise falters, even a small amount of cheating has a large impact. Another point to keep in mind is that the body's reaction to snacking during weight management is so different from the maintenance phase they could be described as different planets. Especially in terms of how the body is responding to the foods that are introduced into it. As long as a person is able to keep up a moderately consistent exercise routine and keep their water intake at 64 ounces per day, the maintenance part of staying lean and healthy is much easier than the weight reduction phase. Yes, keeping the weight off should be easier than dropping the weight. While on the weight maintenance planet, as different as the gravitational pull on the moon is to that on the earth, the comparison can be drawn when it comes to snacking. When you are dropping weight and you have reduced your calorie count, the body goes into a healthy version of starvation mode. This means that a portion of what you eat is converted to glycogen which is stored in your muscles and liver; and then to fat once those glycogen stores are full. When you are in maintenance and you over eat, the fact that you are not in starvation mode means everything, and your body is nowhere near as sensitive to every calorie taken in. Keeping this in mind it is vital that you keep cheating to a minimum as you drop weight. This is explained further in the following weight loss graph of Figure 25.

One thing to think about in terms of snacking is what and where are the situations that make it more likely that you will snack? When actively dropping weight, try not to buy deserts that are already cooked. All deserts need to be the type where preparation is required for you to eat them. This will give you some time to think about what you are doing. If you do cook something tasty that you would normally have a hard time resisting, do not leave it sitting out in the open. Actually tell the family to eat what they want because the rest is going to the neighbor, or a food shelter. One way or the other get that food out of the house.

Many of my patients have told me they find themselves walking into the kitchen for no reason at all. They've told me they will just find themselves staring into the refrigerator. The smart move is to clear out all of the foods that need to be avoided. Stay out of the kitchen unless it is time to cook a meal or prepare a weight management shake etc. Do not keep a television in the kitchen. Do not eat in the living room while watching television. You need to be focusing on your food and how you are feeling as you are eating. When you begin to feel satisfied, stop eating, put the rest in containers and save it for another day.

Ask family members and if you feel comfortable enough, ask co-workers to avoid snacking in front of you. Of course this is only possible if you have let the cat out of the bag as they say and told them that you were on a weight management program. That way they know exactly why you are asking them to do this. Sometimes telling others you are trying to lose weight is the hardest part. This may be because you have had some lack of success in the past. Understand and trust that this time it will be different. What was wrong with you has been addressed medically and you will enjoy nothing but success. The issue of letting people know you are on a weight management program will pop up here and there in the book because of its importance especially in your social circles.

Take the whole weight management program one day at a time. You will not do any of it perfect, (except maybe the water) and your doctor should not expect perfection. Do not be too hard on yourself if you give in to snacking once in a while. It will happen. But the advice I gave you for how to get back to burning fat needs to be followed also. You will find that the longer you stay on track and the more results you see, the easier it will all get. As you stay on track and do your best not only will the weight come off, but you will not have to worry about gaining it back. As long as you are seeing a qualified physician that has diagnosed what was keeping you from reducing weight, you will never need to starve yourself or take part in any fad diets that tend to burn up more muscle than fat. How am I so sure that my program does not burn up muscle? It is because I measure each patients resting metabolic rate at the beginning of the program. I then repeat this test after they complete the weight management and transition phases.

Figure 25: Weight Management Medicine Graph

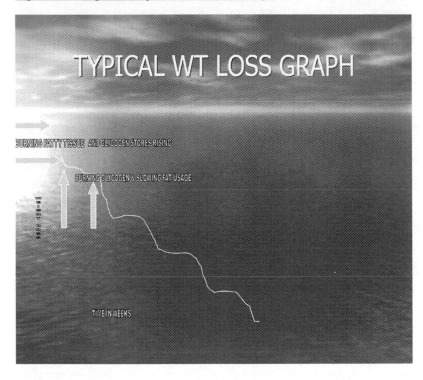

The weight management graph above is one that you would typically see if you pulled 8 out of 10 of my medical charts. I call this the "Weight management Stair Step Graph" of progress. I have explained what you are looking at in different parts of the book, but it makes more sense hopefully when you see it. When I see a graph that looks like this, showing 3-5 pounds of weight reduction per week, I know things are going well. If you were to draw a line right down the middle of the graph, it would be a steep line. The steeper the line the faster the person whose graph it represents is reducing their weight.

By way of further explanation, the graphed portion between the vertical arrows represents those times when you are burning stored glycogen primarily. Yes, even the small amount of carbohydrates that are present on my programs is enough for our bodies to store and use for energy around every other week. The body is burning fat also, albeit small amounts and from the abdominal region in most instances. This is why people will experience a drop in their waistline in the absence of a significant drop in pounds. The graphed portion between the horizontal arrows represents a drop in fatty tissue with an accompanying decrease in pounds on the scale. DO NOT WEIGH YOURSELF EVERY DAY while on an active weight management program. It will only serve to drive you completely nuts! I have my patients drink 64 ounces of at rest water per day. Water is the gasoline that drives weight management and burning fat is absolutely dependant on this water intake. Drink half the amount of water and you will only lose half the amount of weight. All of that water you drink daily is shifting around your body. One day you may weigh yourself when you have burned fat over the previous seven days and water has been used by your body globally. Your weight will be most likely down and that is good. However, on a different day you may find that when you weigh yourself you have caught your body at a time when this fat has not been burned yet. In this situation your body will still be holding on to that water because you have weighed yourself smack in the middle of burning fat and you will weigh heavy, or weigh the same. Seven days is about the minimum I have found that I can get an accurate view of how well a person is doing over a given amount of time. I could weigh everyone every 10 days, but every 7 days seems to work out well for scheduling purposes.

The previous graph represents what I call the "Dichotomy of Weight Management". This is when the patient loses weight on the scale, but their abdominal girth goes up or stays the same. I believe this is because of what I mentioned above regarding the use of water for weight management. When we measure the abdominal girth and it is the same and yet the person has lost 4 pounds, they are quite confused. The answer is that the body is holding onto water in the abdomen and using it to help drive many of the chemical reactions that help turn triglycerides (the storage form of fat) into free fatty acids. These fatty acids are then transported out of the fat cell and excreted in the feces or used by the muscles during exercise. On the other days, the abdominal girth may reduce 2 inches and the patient only loses 1-2 pounds. This is the body holding onto water globally as fatty tissue is being burned all over the body. The scale will go up and down all week. This is why I advise against weighing yourself daily.

I try to warn all of my patients about the second week of weight management. I call the second week of weight management "The Second Week Evolutionary Slowdown". I tell men and women that there is very little they can do about this slow down. This is a response to what your body considers a famine, or, at the very least, a serious decrease in the amount of "available food in the cave." For a few agonizing days the body burns very little fat and burns glycogen stores instead. Patients also report that they feel fatigued and hungrier than the first week. It is easy to understand when explained another way. What is the best way for the body to try and ensure that you do not burn calories if there is a shortage of food? The answer is to keep you sitting on your couch and basically burn as few calories as possible. If the patient is able to resist this urge to sit around and eat, but instead exercises and controls their food intake, they will be fine. Weight will fluctuate very little during this second week. I have seen this second week slow down occur in the third week. If it does not happen by the third week then it may not happen at all. The reason I bring this up is because some people begin to feel as though the program is not working for them. So take this paragraph to heart and remember to push through this short time and the weight reduction will pick back up. There are many issues that need to be addressed in a weight management program. For the majority of the population it will always be more complex than just "calories in and calories out".

POW: IF YOU HAVE MORE CALORIES THAN YOU WERE SUPPOSED TO ON A GIVEN DAY, DO NOT CUT BACK ON CALORIES THE NEXT DAY. GET BACK ON YOUR PROGRAM AND ACCOUNT FOR THOSE EXTRA CALORIES WITH ADDITIONAL EXERCISE.

Support:

The first and most important point I want to bring up regarding this issue is not leaving the fact that you are trying to lose weight a secret. What would be the main reason you would keep this VERY large part of your life hidden from everyone? The answer is somewhat depressing, because it borders on an admission of failure before it even becomes an issue. Is it possible that you are afraid of failing and the more people you tell the more people will know if you do? Because the only reason people fail to lose weight on one of my programs is if they just quit.

On the flip side the more people you tell the more support you have. I would like to think that a dedicate doctor is all anyone would need to be successful. But having a husband or wife that is there supporting you is invaluable. Behind every successful athlete there is usually a good coach and family. Yes it is true that when you go out to dinner with friends and family eyes may be on you that are discriminating what you are putting in your mouth. In the end though isn't that what you really need. Everyone talks about needing accountability to be successful. Well the ultimate accountability is to the people that are around you practically 24/7. You will only see the doctor at most once per week, and if you really want to you can lie to him or her. It's tough to lie to your son as he walks into the kitchen and sees you sticking a cookie in your mouth. Besides, these are the people you love and aside from yourself, are probably the ones you are doing this for. You want to be able to play with your children or grandchildren and not have to stop after 10 minutes because you're too out of breath.

Believe with every fiber of your being that you can get this done. Believe your doctor is going to find out what is wrong with you and approach weight reduction as a team. I tell women and men that if they are even a little bit "OK with being overweight" they are not ready to get started. I want people that are totally committed to accepting all of the support I want them to enlist in this process of weight management. I do not care how much pressure it puts on them "because so many people know" what they are doing. It will only serve to help them stick a little closer to what I want them to do. One thing is for sure you cannot do it alone. I would even go as far as to say that when your doctor is the only person "in the know", you are very close to doing it alone. Sometimes a person is single or there are simply circumstances that are in place where any more support than that is impossible. If that is the case the patient and I do our best and we work through it. But if more people can be enlisted in this process of weight management then I advise my patients to have them climb aboard!

It is important that you pick the right sort of people for support. You surely cannot expect support from those who are not even aware you are trying to drop weight. They will continue to offer you food that is unhealthy, and in amounts that are way above your allowed limit. They cannot be blamed though, they don't know any better. You may find yourself eating what they serve so you don't hurt their feelings. If this person is a good friend then telling them should be first priority so they can have a chance to adjust to the new you. You'll find yourself getting angry with them for making the weight management process so hard if you don't tell them. You may even find that once you get the weight off and then tell them how hard it was coming over to their house for dinners they get extremely upset. So you may want to think twice in regards to who you tell you're trying to lose weight. They certainly don't want to think back to all of those invites and realize that you may have dreaded coming over because of the fear that they were contributing to your early demise from serving food you would have rather not eaten.

On the flip side, laying too much responsibility on just one person is not such a good idea either. Saying to a friend "I want you to help me lose weight" may be a little too much to lay on a friend who for years has known you as the person who eats and acts in a completely different way. It would be more appropriate to ask each person to take on specific responsibilities. For instance it may be one friend's job to make sure you have gotten in enough water for the day. This needs to be a pretty reliable person because remember, when attempting to adhere to "The Ashworth Weigh" there is only one thing I want all of my patients to attempt to perform perfectly, drinking water.

As I have said over and over exercise is one of the most important components of any weight management program and especially weight maintenance programs. The person you pick to be your support person for exercise needs to be someone who already exercises regularly. Someone who will be there at the specified time, possibly call you and will walk whether you go or not. You don't want someone who struggles with exercise already. This is a person who may not go exercise if you do not exercise, then both of you will be hindered. What you do want though is for that person to feel completely comfortable asking you where you were. And you cannot get mad or defensive at any of these people. You enlisted them to support you and they need to feel comfortable trying to hold you responsible for the things you say you will and will not do. Make sure to enlist someone who simply will listen. They do not necessarily work on giving advice or fixing a problem they just listen and tell you that they understand.

One person that definitely needs to be on board is your spouse. Your spouse must support your new eating habits. One way he or she can do this is by not bringing things into the house that you are not supposed to eat like pizza, ice cream, candy, etc. If possible he or she may even try to eat the same dinners you prepare for yourself. The dinners you eat on a healthy weight management program should be a part of most people's menus anyhow. Things like steak, pork, chicken, and fish is a commonly served entrée in most households. The one or two things he or she may have to sacrifice being on the table are things like rice, breads, or potatoes. The thing to remember and to remind the spouse of is that this is only for a limited amount of time. That is something I tell my patients often, **you do not have to do this forever!** Managing your health as you reduce weight is just one part of a completely different way of living. One thing to tell your spouse for sure is to never reward you for hard work and successful weight management with more food like deserts and the like. Non-food rewards are the key in this department. These may include a day at the spa, massages, or clothing.

Secondly, spouses are of monumental importance in the area of exercise. There is nothing like having your own workout partner living with you. This is because both of you know and understand the others schedule. If things still need to get done in the house or you had to work late the spouse will understand and will not look at it as an excuse as may someone outside of the family.

Remember, <u>none of these people you are recruiting as your support group are mind readers</u>. Unless you tell them what you are looking for and what the goals are you are trying to accomplish how will they know? Once people know you want help, most of the time they are more than willing to lend a hand. The problem is that some of their help may not be helpful at all. If what they are trying to do is hurtful instead of helpful, tell them. You need to make sure to communicate your goals to everyone involved in this journey. If they don't know you're trying to change you can't get mad at them if they treat you like the person you are trying desperately not to be anymore.

It may be surprising at how some of your friends and family react to you as you succeed. The one thing I will say for sure is try and be patient with them. They are not used to this new person, this slender person with a new attitude. Especially if some of your friends or family is still overweight or tried something different and were unsuccessful. This is especially true of your spouse if they are overweight. They may become quite jealous of your nights out with the girls, or a night out with the guys. Give them time to adjust and to understand all of the positive reasons you lost the weight. If they are sparked by your success and give it the "good college try" to drop weight they have you to thank. Always try to remember the struggles you went through, because it may just be you they enlist for support.

As the number of people grows that you tell your goals to, it may be surprising who informs you they had also been overweight. They usually have a lot of advice to offer on how to get the job done successfully. You may be lucky enough to find someone in the middle of the weight management process looking for people like yourself to help motivate and support them. One point is for sure though; if you decide to not let a single sole know what you are trying to accomplish none of these people you might meet will be around. Who knows, your attitude may initiate a chain reaction where others decide to start exercising or eating right. Positive attitudes just like negative ones are contagious. But beware there will always be naysayers and those that will try and throw you off track. When conversations you are involved in start to lead to negative comments, either leave or try to redirect the focus of the conversation.

Emotional support is very important. It is even more important to understand that what may be a weakness to you may not be a weakness to someone else. I like my patients to have a person they are trying to lose weight with, a "buddy system" if you will. This system can be more complicated than it might first appear. In essence there are two types of buddy systems, one the "Shared Weakness System", the other is the "Unshared Weakness System". Which of the two systems a pair chooses depends on how they each historically handle temptation and motivation? Some people feel as though they react better to those they can relate to when it comes to resisting temptations. Shared experiences, successes and failures allow these types to help each other through common histories of dealing with the same problems. The other types would rather be around another person that has strength where they may be weak. They are motivated by others that may have "already been there" or can offer advice on what turned that area into strength for them. So it is important to choose your partners in weight management wisely.

> **POW:** *DO NOT HIDE THE FACT THAT YOU ARE TRYING TO DROP WEIGHT FROM YOUR FRIENDS AND FAMILY JUST BECAUSE OF A FEAR OF FAILING. USE THE SUPPORT THESE PEOPLE OFFER AND TAKE RESPONSIBILITY FOR YOUR DECISION TO GET HEALTHY.*

Motivation and reasonable Thinking:

There are basically two different types of motivators; those that talk very harshly to themselves and those that are a bit kinder. The first group tends to concentrate on the negative, leaning more towards rebellion and self victimization. They live in the past. The other is the person who takes a gentler approach, understands that they are in a program that has worked for many people and will also work for them. They try to use words like "I Choose To", "I Want To" which are more empowering. Every day is going to require some sort of change, some new angle of approach in this journey towards changing the way you look at yourself and what constitutes health.

Who are you losing the weight for? It needs to be for you, because I have found those people to be the most successful. It is most commonly called being internally motivated. Most of the patients in my programs flip flop between accepting and resisting the process of changing. The key to all of this is to understand and believe it will work and not QUIT. Try your best to be kind to yourself and be **your own best friend,** which is certainly an internal motivation. There will be many people out there to tear you down. You certainly do not need to be one of them. There will be many times when you will be weak and indulge in something you shouldn't. It's not the end of the world or certainly the program, just get back on track the next day. In the case of reducing weight it is always better to take 3 steps forward and 1 step back; than to take 1 step back get discouraged because you're not perfect and quit. So, don't try to be a perfectionist! When you try and be a perfectionist, knowing good and well that you will never be one, it may be a sign that you are beginning to resist the changes that it will take to make the program work for you. Think rationally, none of us walking this earth is perfect.

What I have every person do when they come into my clinic is write down ten reasons why they want to lose weight. At the time they are writing down those ten reasons they are feeling very motivational thoughts, and are trying to prepare themselves to change certain behaviors. When you are feeling weak, this is the time to pull out those reasons and re-read each of them slowly trying to recapture what you were feeling at that time. This is the time to recognize the mood you are currently in or events that have occurred in your life that led you to resisting the urge to lose the weight. Once you recognize those moods or events try to face them directly. Share them with your doctor so you can receive some advice and support. If a top 10 reason is to change the way your body looks, have a friend take a Polaroid of you front and back. Glue them together and keep them with you all the time in your wallet or in your purse. When you are feeling weak go into the bathroom take out that picture and remind yourself why you got started. It sounds harsh but in a lot of cases it works fairly well.

Another idea is to purchase a small recorder and record yourself talking about those 10 reasons why you want to lose weight. You may also want to continue to use this audio taping as a sort of weight management journal. A journal where you write down what happened and how you performed the week before. I also find that my written thoughts, especially if I am tired are briefer and less detailed. Talk about why those reasons are so important. Or of course replay the recorded reasons you wanted to lose weight that I suggested above. Either way they represent you at a certain point in your life that led you to make the decision to start a weight management program. Getting started is the hardest part for some. Being able to listen to the level of motivation you had when you first started may be just the thing to keep you going in the middle of the weight management process.

It may sound ridiculous but the last topic I bring up when I am trying to motivate a person is health concerns that arise from remaining obese. But in fact it is fairly difficult for me to motivate a person to stay on a program based on health conditions alone. If it is later in the program and I've already got them off of their diabetic injections that is a bit more powerful as a motivator to stay on track. The idea of going to the pharmacy again once per month and picking up syringes and needles; and then injecting themselves daily <u>again</u> is a pretty strong deterrent to quitting.

Wishful thinking will not get the job done. Just because you really want something to happen does not mean that it will. Honestly ask yourself what you are willing and not willing to do in order to drop the weight. After talking with your doctor and finding out what it will take, write down a concrete list of actions and behaviors in order of importance. Talking and talking about the "intention" of doing it does not get it done—get committed! You have to believe that you can get it done. You have to have the self confidence; the sense of ability that you can accomplish this job of changing your lifestyle and getting all of the weight off.

One time a woman told me "You know why you are so successful at helping people lose weight". I didn't answer because that was a very gracious thing to say; I just asked her why she thought I was. She said "It's because when you look at me you see the person that is inside, the healthier more slender and confident person that I want to be". That was the first time I had considered what it was that might have allowed me to connect so quickly with my patients. I seem to see and talk to the person in that patient's *"mind's eye"*. They know it and can feel it very early on in the conversation. Having said this I would like to point out that it is critical for you to accept the person you are right now. This is because the person you are RIGHT NOW, not the healthier, slender one in 90 days or 9 months; the one you see in the mirror, that is the person that needs to get the job done. Notice though I still emphasize getting the job done. You will never read that I am fine with people being overweight or obese. As a physician it would be unethical for me or any doctor to advocate a body fat percent that results in so many disease processes.

There are a couple of groups that advocate the acceptance of people that are of a "large stature". The problem is that in most cases these organizations tend to delay the time to treatment that people take to get the weight off. If being obese or overweight failed to lead to all of the disorders numerous studies have shown they do that stance might be acceptable. I certainly agree that people of large stature should not be discriminated against in the work place or socially. The problem I have is when these associations fail to recognize all of the health problems being overweight or obese causes. I support an absence of discrimination across the board. But right along with this these organizations need to offer their members smart ways to help them understand the importance of reducing their weight to more healthy levels. If they fail in this area, and focus solely on convincing people that it is fine being obese, these organizations are worthless.

Never base yourself worth on the fact that you happen to be overweight. For one thing the condition you are in is like the name of this book, a condition that may not even be your fault. On top of that it will be a short term condition once you meet the correct physician that is willing to get the job done correctly. You have to believe strongly in your ability to change things that may need changing. As often as you can, try to keep company with positive people that tend to build you up, motivate and make you feel good about yourself, and the changes you want to make. Negative people can really sap your energy. Try to spend as little time as possible with these people. Our goal is to try and think as rationally as possible. Try and remember this motto from the Ashworth coat of arms: **"Appetitus rationi pareat"**. The english translation reads: **"Let your desires obey your reason"**.

Changing the way you think can be difficult when you may have lived the first 18 years with parents that encouraged you to always clean your plate of food. When serving sizes are now 20% larger in restaurants than they used to be, eating every bit of your food on the plate can pile on the calories. You have to get to a place where you understand how your body feels, and what that body is trying to tell you. If you feel satisfied with what you have eaten then feel free to leave the rest alone and take it home. The only caveat being that you have worked your way around the plate and eaten all of the foods that are nutritious in the correct amounts. You can always eat what is left on the plate the next day. It may even be a good idea once you have become accustomed to what your portions are supposed to look like to just have the server take a portion of the meal away and simply bag it up at the beginning of a meal. This will need you to change the way you look at eating out. It isn't fair to your spouse to tell them you are no longer allowed to eat out. You should still try to keep those important date nights. The focus will just need to change from how much food you get for the price, to the casual conversation you can enjoy with the person you are out with that night.

POW: UNDERSTAND THAT YOUR ENTHUSIASM FOR DROPPING WEIGHT WILL WAX AND WANE. WHEN YOU START OUT WRITE DOWN OR RECORD YOUR VOICE AS YOU SHARE 10 REASONS YOU WANT TO GET THE WEIGHT OFF. READ OR LISTEN TO THESE REASONS WHENEVER YOU FEEL LIKE YOU ARE SLIPPING.

Eating out:

A generation or so ago it was more of a special event when a family went out to dinner together. Now the whole feeling of eating out has changed to an event that is not a question of if, but when and where on any given day. One unfortunate part of this is the fast food industry and the increasing role they play in the decisions families make as they decide to eat out. It is certainly encouraging that a few large fast food chains have begun to offer more healthy options for children. The best option in the long run will always be to avoid these establishments as often as possible.

When people choose to eat out during a weight management program they are taking a chance on the way the food is prepared and what the ingredients and sauces are the restaurant uses. The only way to ensure the food is prepared properly is to call ahead and see if the chef is accustomed to taking special orders. Go to a number of restaurants and get their menus so you know ahead of time what they have to order. Some restaurants have heart healthy selections. It will also help with budgeting money each week. Most people will find that weight management programs where medical shakes are part of the program actually will save them money each month, because eating out can be expensive.

When we are faced with a lot of eating out opportunities we need to try and classify them. When we classify them, we can better prepare a plan of action for how we are going to conduct ourselves. When you are taking part in a weight management program this is the time to try and skip as many non-necessity eating out opportunities as possible. Business lunches or dinners are sometimes a required part of the job for marketing executives, to name just one. Stress is usually going to be involved and stress can make you want to let your guard down so go in prepared. As prepared as you try to be in whatever presentation you must give or listen to; this is the same level of preparation you want to put into how you are going to eat. Attorneys (my wife being one) are notorious for wanting to have lunch. They can literally find any excuse in the world to go out and eat. Bringing a new attorney into the practice, go out to lunch. Want to meet the expert in the field, go out to lunch. Want to introduce your daughter, who just graduated from law school to the heavy hitters in the community, go out to lunch. Hey its Friday . . . go out to lunch.

When eating out for celebrations like birthdays or weddings, these events are always associated with food, but you do not *necessarily* have to eat. Everyone knows if you want a high attendance rate for a church activity serve food. When you know one of these events are on the schedule for the day try to eat prior to the event. This is when the use of medically engineered shakes can come in handy.

Figure 26: A Few Rules When Eating Out For Business

- Do a lot of talking, not hard if you are presenting at a business meeting
- Take a drink of water in between each bite
- Make sure you do not drink too much alcohol before ordering your main meal, it lowers inhibitions
- Put your fork down in between each bite
- If eating a salad have the dressing on the side, and dip the fork in the dressing *prior to* spearing the salad bite
- Keep the carbohydrate enriched breads either off the table or on the other side of the table

If appropriate tell the people at the meeting that you are trying to lose a few pounds and this is why you seem to be eating so little or slowly, not because the food tastes bad.

This will make it easier to go lighter on the food that is served. So the word for these types of events is personal planning. You can be assured that peer pressure will be in effect at these gatherings. There will be a general sense of "cutting loose" and going past normal boundaries. Certain people might stress you out. Try to avoid these people if possible because stress can lead to bad decisions when choosing what and how much to consume. The above rules can be applied in either the business or casual situations.

Just understand that in this situation of eating out, whether for business or family, change will be required. Try to avoid buffets or "all you can eat" specialty night restaurants. Ok do not try to avoid buffets, avoid buffets. This will be especially critical during the active weight reduction phase. It may sound funny but rehearse what you are going to say to those people that are going to pressure you to eat more than you are planning to. Part of that planning will include what you are going to do to make up for those extra calories that may be eaten. From what has already been written we know that starving yourself the night before or after is more damaging than helpful. When you play, you pay. The way you pay is by exercising a bit more on the day before and after. You do not cut your calories the day before or after, just stick with the program and add in a few more minutes of exercise. Whatever calorie count you are on when reducing weight will be the lowest amount to lower your weight in the shortest yet healthiest way. If you begin taking it upon yourself to lower or change the eating regimen you were put on by your doctor you're headed for trouble.

When looking at the acronym FIT; Frequency, Intensity, and Time, it should be the intensity and the time that are adjusted to a more difficult level. You will get a feel as to how much to adjust these based on how your body responds. Everyone is different as I've said over and over, and it will take learning and listening to your body the days that follow these episodes of over eating that will tell you.

For family related eating out, or a date with your spouse instead of concentrating on how good the food is going to be, consider a couple of other activities you would have ended up doing if you were not eating out. There is no cooking involved by you, and no dishes to be washed afterwards. You can take advantage of relaxed conversation, and the well deserved time away from the children in an enjoyable environment. The take home point of this is just because you have decided to lose weight does not mean you need to completely avoid eating out; just change how it is approached. Eating out still needs to be an event you look forward to not feared, even when you are on a weight management program.

POW: WHEN EATING OUT TAKE A DRINK OF WATER IN BETWEEN EACH BITE, EAT SLOWLY, SET YOUR FORK DOWN IN BETWEEN BITES, TALK A LOT, AND SIMPLY ENJOY THE ATMOSPHERE AND PERSON YOU ARE WITH INSTEAD OF MAKING THE FOOD THE SOLE FOCUS.

Stress:

One of the most common responses I get when I ask a patient how their week went is "it was a stressful week". This can be translated to "LIFE occurred this week and I responded to LIFE the way I have prior to coming here and I do not desire to hear from you how to better deal with this thing called LIFE. Leave me alone you're lucky I even showed up to my appointment today. Actually, just give me my shakes and get out of my way". All of us experience stress. Actually life would probably be a bit boring without a little stress. Since stress is involved with goal attainment and the old adage "nothing worth having comes easy" is probably true in most cases. So, accepting that stress is not going anywhere all that is left is how we reduce and then deal with what is left. There are a lot of people out there who deal with stress by eating, turning to what they refer to as comfort foods. It's important to remember that stress is not an event or a situation, but how we deal with the stressor. For some it may manifest itself as a simple panicky feeling. Others may have a global increase in all systems like breathing and heart rate to name just a couple. Something is only stressful when we perceive it to be. Flying a jet aircraft at mach 3 might be perceived as stressful to many people. Being a trauma surgeon might be the same situation. Yet the men and women who choose these as their careers see them for the most part as anything but stressful.

If stress is experienced over the long term the immune system may begin to break down. We find ourselves getting sick easier. We find ourselves feeling like we have an overall lack of energy to perform the simplest of tasks. Some people turn to food because they say it makes them feel good. It is a proven fact that food can actually increase certain chemicals in the brain that give a sense of calmness as discussed earlier. The problem is that it is very temporary; and the food has to be eaten again and again, and in larger amounts akin to medications that people can become resistant to, and subsequently addicted to.

There are different types of stressors and people respond differently to them. Everyone needs to identify their own life stressors and more importantly how they deal with those stressors. There are many different types of stressors, those that affect you from the inside and those from the outside. There are those that are short term and longer term stressors to deal with. The most common outside stressors are poor working environments and abusive relationships. Those that affect the inside are mostly physiologic in nature and include infection and inflammation.

One stressor that I have found avoidable if my patients would listen to a little advice is the stress from weighing themselves daily during active weight reduction. Remember *weight can fluctuate up to 5 pounds in one day!* We retain and lose water daily from hour to hour. The only time it is OK to weigh yourself daily is when you are in the maintenance phase weight management. Then you are able to see trends as they occur and catch something you may be doing wrong before it gets too out of hand. But do not weigh yourself daily during active weight reduction because it creates a small fight or flight response every time you hop on that scale. I tell my patients to weigh themselves once per week when they are in an active weight reduction phase and when at the clinic to see their doctor.

This world we live in produces an environment where it seems there is always some sort of stress to be dealt with. This sort of ongoing chronic stress is unhealthy. It releases hormones that hinder weight management and makes weight gain easier. All of this stress triggers the release of steroid hormones, namely cortisol. This type of hormone along with other fight or flight hormones are usually burned off once the threat is gone. A crude, evolutionary example of this would be seeing a bear that then sees you which triggers the release of all of these hormones, allowing you to start sprinting. In our daily lives we are releasing these stress hormones like cortisol and not burning them off. There is something to the adage "Stress is a killer". If we do not exercise and effectively burn off these stress hormones, they just continue to build. This becomes a persistent state that you live in where your major organs like brain, heart, and blood vessels become chronically over or under activated. This produces both physical and psychological damage. You absolutely, positively have to exercise. Not just to reduce weight more quickly, effectively, and permanently, but to keep you alive and feeling like you want to be alive after the weight is gone by controlling stress levels.

Specifically, certain neurotransmitters in our brains change their levels when under stress, these few go up: epinephrine, norepinephrine and histamine. Serotonin can either go up or down, but as stated we do know that cortisol will go up in an attempt to reduce anxiety and stress. Cortisol is supposed to do this by decreasing epinephrine and norepinephrine. Cortisol also increases GABA receptors which is an attempt to reduce neurotransmitter activity, thus having a calming effect. DHEA goes up in an attempt to enhance serotonin and norepinephrine; therefore it can have a calming or excitatory effect.

Numerous studies have suggested that the inability to adapt to stress is associated with the onset of depression and anxiety. Actually the inability to adapt to chronic stressors makes a person six times as likely to become depressed. These studies have suggested that the stress causes hyperactivity in the brain which diminishes the supply over time of serotonin. Serotonin is involved with the feeling of well being. This obviously decreases a person's quality of life, along with their relationships with their mate or co-workers.

Stress and the subsequent anxiety and depression can adversely affect the heart. With the release of all of these hormones that tend to stimulate the body, people can experience chest pain and irregular rhythms of the heart. When I say stimulates the body I am talking about increasing the activity of the sympathetic nervous system. This in turn can cause the heart to beat faster and the blood pressure to go up; these hormones can also cause the blood to become thicker which increases the chances of an artery clogging blood clot. Stress can also trigger the body to release fat into the blood stream. When people lead sedentary lifestyles and this fat is not burned off it can lead to high cholesterol levels.

This is beginning to look a lot like a well known syndrome sweeping the country as the number of overweight, untreated people rise, "Metabolic Syndrome" or "Syndrome X".

> **Figure 27: Metabolic Syndrome or Syndrome X**
> - Elevated blood pressure
> - Increased abdominal girth which goes along with being overweight or obese
> - Small vessel artery disease
> - Elevated sugar levels, and elevated insulin levels
> - Elevated triglycerides, and in many cases an overall increase in cholesterol levels

These sorts of symptoms and the inability to appropriately deal with stress can cause people to habitually eat when they feel the stress coming on. They may begin to crave carbohydrates and fats. The majority of this seems to be in response to elevated levels of the hormone mentioned above cortisol. The weight gain that is most prominent when triggered by cortisol is in the abdominal region. The bad news is that studies have shown that there are very few if any pills that by themselves decrease cortisol levels. Especially if the way we deal with stress or the main stressor is not removed from the situation. The next paragraph could very well be the most important one in this book. It deals with one of the primary areas of medicine where I feel a paradigm shift is in order as to how the medical community deals with diabetes.

We know that the abdominal fat termed *visceral adipose tissue* (fat that is under your abdominal muscles and around your organs) releases the hormone *Resistin* which renders the person resistant to the affects of insulin. This molecule is released from fat cells in the abdomen whether stress is controlled or not. In other words once the weight is gained and the fat is present in this area the release of Resistin is set in motion. The next logical question is how does Resistin affect the body so adversely? As abdominal fat increases, Resistin as well as a multitude of other inflammatory mediators are released in larger amounts. In response to this the body has to produce more insulin to get the sugar levels down to where they were before the weight was gained. When the person goes to their doctor and has a simple fasting sugar level measured it may come out normal! HOWEVER this is only because the poor pancreas is working so hard pumping out insulin to keep the sugar levels normal. Eventually the pancreas cannot produce enough insulin to lower the sugars, and finally the diagnosis of type II diabetes is made. In reality the "diabetic" condition has been there for quite a while (probably years) taking its toll on the body. Insulin in high levels in the blood makes it difficult if not nearly impossible to lose weight as I have stated before. And yet early on the sugar level is normal and all looks well. The trick is to dig deeper medically and measure the levels of fasting insulin in the blood, start to lower insulin by increasing insulin sensitivity and get the weight off before damage to the pancreas occurs. I realize this was written about in the diabetes section but the importance of the hormone insulin and how and when it is tested for and reduced can never be overemphasized.

Going back to stress, what are some healthy ways we can start to decrease our stress, or at least learn how to deal with it better? It is simply imperative that we learn to lower stress because cortisol is no friend to weight management. For most people we simply cannot remove the stressors from our lives like our job or raising children or dealing with in-laws. Instead we need to come up with novel ways to help ourselves relax more. Some ideas will work for one person and not work at all for another. When trying certain activities out listen to your body, does your mind relax a bit more during the activity or do the opposite? In other words the activity needs to make you feel physically good while you are doing it or after you've done it. Something else to consider is to make lists of the activities and or people that affect you in positive or negative ways. Try to increase or decrease the daily contact with these people and or situations as much as possible. This will help decrease the daily release of those stress hormones.

I have always been a big advocate of daily exercise, or at a minimum four days per week of some sort of exercise done for at least thirty minutes. This is the healthiest approach to burning off those stress hormones. Schedule yourself a weekly or bi-weekly massage. This is also something that I advocate and enjoy. If you haven't had a vacation in a while it is probably high time you tried to take one. It could be something as simple as a long weekend where you take a Friday or Monday off and play. Everyone needs recreation or activities that they enjoy doing in their off time, which you need to schedule into your life! I love surfing and mixed martial arts and do both as often as my schedule will permit.

Women who are "stay at home moms" need to have days or weeks when they allocate the chores of the household to other members of the family. Your only responsibility will be to relax and find new and interesting ways to cut down on stress. Sometimes just going out for a bike ride on a beautiful day is enough. This will not even necessarily be a ride for exercise, just a ride to get out of the house.

Deep breathing exercises are always a good idea because as we become stressed our breathing usually becomes shallow and rapid. You inhale through the nose slowly counting to ten, making sure that the chest does not rise, but that the abdomen expands. Exhale to a count of ten through the nose, trying very hard to concentrate on the breathing and counting. Muscle relaxation is also a way to unwind where you lie down in a comfortable position without crossing any limbs. Maintain a nice slow breathing pattern. Starting with your head you tense each muscle as tightly as possible for a count of five and then release it completely. Try to imagine the muscle as totally relaxed and lead-heavy after releasing it.

Do not keep the fact that you are overly stressed to yourself. Make sure to tell those closest to you how you are feeling. It may surprise you what they are willing to do to help you relax. I have kept a journal since 1995, writing down my daily activities and thoughts. I have found this to be a great way to unwind and identify which aspects of your life give you the most misery or satisfaction. Looking at Adrenal Fatigue after long episodes of life stressors or chronic illness is a good idea and needs to be brought up to your physician because as stated in the hormone section, adrenal fatigue will diminish your quality of life as you get into your mid-life years.

Another problem I catch women and men doing is obsessing over the weight management. I try to tell them there is a reason I have been able to stay in the business of helping people lose weight for so long; and it is because if they will relax and let me do my job the weight will come off. If a patient is a referral I try to remind them of the weight their friend lost and how they can expect the same. But 9 times out of 10 they are obsessing and sometimes weighing themselves not just daily, but multiple times per day. Try to remember; you came to the clinic for a reason so take the advice of the physician you have trusted!

This seems like a perfect place to write about the stress relieving benefits of **massage therapy**. There are many benefits to a massage aside from decreasing stress of which I am a huge advocate. With any weight management program you are going to need to exercise and massage therapy improves flexibility which in turn increases endurance and shortens recovery time. Massage also reduces the risk of injury by stretching connective tissue, improving circulation, and influencing the excretion of toxins and breakdown products from weight management.

If you have heard that massage therapy increases metabolism it is true. It accomplishes this through the increase in the supply of nutrients and oxygen as the blood and lymph flow is improved. It is vital to understand that the more oxygen your body has for use, the better the metabolic rate will be. Of course as you decrease stress through massage you will decrease the release of cortisol, which as I wrote earlier helps weight management. Massage will also increase tonicity and skin elasticity that is required as patients lose weight and are trying to avoid loose skin. But in the end it rewards dedication and hard work as you improve the look and health of your body through a healthy weight management program.

POW: *NEVER DOUBT THAT STRESS IS A KILLER. ONE EASY STEP TO TAKE ON CUTTING DOWN ON THIS KILLER IS TO AVOID WEIGHING YOURSELF EVERY DAY DURING THE ACTIVE WEIGHT MANAGEMENT PHASE. ONCE PER WEEK IS THE FREQUENCY TO SHOOT FOR.*

Food addictions:

Many of my patients tell me that they seem to be addicted to chocolate. Actually I've had patients tell me they are addicted to a whole range of foods. There is a scientific reason for these food addictions. Many foods have an opiate effect, yes opiates like those found in addictive narcotic pain medications. Chocolate has quite a bit of a chemical called phenylethylamine which is an amphetamine-like substance. Once chocolate is eaten brain cells release a chemical called anandamide, which is related to THC (associated with marijuana). Chocolate is actually able to delay the breakdown of anandamide which prolongs the opiate like effects felt when chocolate is eaten. So chocolate can be quite addictive as many foods can be. Not as addictive as the drugs we have come to know like cocaine or alcohol, but for many eating certain foods is extremely difficult to resist. An addictive behavior is one that when indulged in repeatedly results in diminished health, job performance or advancement, and in social relationships. In spite of the negative consequences, if the behavior is continued it is officially an addiction.

Cheese and dairy products contain the same sort of chemicals as chocolate. Cheese contains the protein casein, when casein is broken down the opiates that are released from these foods are referred to as casomorphins (resembles the word morphine). So when patients say they do not know if they can give up their milk and cheese it is no big surprise. I'm not going to spend a lot of time going over all of the foods that are addictive. I just wanted you the reader to know that I understand that yes, you very well may be addicted to this or that type of food for very specific reasons. But in reality there are many chemicals and products made that can be addictive and we should try to avoid them. You can do the same with food, you need to find a doctor and work as a team to find out the best approach to beating the addiction. As far as I am concerned it is the doctor's job to make his or her patient aware of which foods are addictive and steer their patients' away from them. I will admit that I put a lot of responsibility squarely on the shoulders of the physicians out there. This is because we are in the midst of what is being called an epidemic of obesity and patients need physicians that are as well informed as possible.

> *POW: SINCE NONE OF US CAN EVER ABSTAIN FROM FOOD COMPLETELY, IT IS IMPORTANT TO CULTIVATE A HEALTHY RELATIONSHIP WITH FOOD FROM THE BEGINNING OF ANY PROGRAM.*

CHAPTER 12

I am Inflamed and Allergic to Food

Inflammatory Hormones:

The old theory that fatty tissue primarily served as a storage depot has been proven untrue. In fact inflammation and being overweight go hand in hand. Cortisol is sent out by the adrenals to deal with stress, but just like cortisol when our bodies are exposed to inflammation too long it becomes unhealthy and causes disease. First we will discuss how fatty tissues along with all of the inflammatory mediators that are released from it affect Leptin. Leptin normally serves as a signal to the brain that there has been adequate food intake to allow fat storage and subsequently lets a person begin to feel full. Leptin then sets up a cascade of activities that is supposed to begin burning this fat for energy working in conjunction with insulin. It has been discovered that a certain percent of people are resistant to the affects of Leptin.

Simply being obese can lower the levels of Leptin. Having too much intake of sugars in general can lower levels of Leptin. As we lose weight we become more sensitive to the signals of Leptin along with being more sensitive to the levels of insulin. As one loses weight, especially the weight stored inside the abdominal cavity, insulin resistance drops which then allows Leptin levels to rise and perform the job of telling the brain you do not need any additional storage of fatty tissue. Leptin levels are also affected by levels of cholesterol and triglycerides; as they drop, Leptin levels are allowed to rise naturally. So as you continue to see, this whole issue of having an over abundance of fat on your body is far reaching and affects a multitude of healthy as well as unhealthy hormonal signals.

Another hormone worthy of mention is adiponectin. The job of this hormone among many is to lower sugar levels and raise our sensitivity to insulin. It also helps us keep our arteries cleaner, and plaque free. This is a natural hormone created in our body designed to help us stay healthy. For those of us who would rather not take medicines for diabetes and high cholesterol we would not need to if we would work to keep our weight under control. There are biological mechanisms in place to help us control the majority of conditions that we spend billions of dollars to "keep under control" using very expensive medications. We know that inflammatory mediators released by fatty tissue like Interleukin-6, Interleukin-1, and tumor necrosis factor alpha along with chronic increases in epinephrine (adrenalin) all decrease the levels of adiponectin. It becomes more obvious why we feel so lousy when we are carrying extra fat on our bodies.

An additional hormone that fat cells cause release of is Acylation Stimulating Protein (ASP). When we gain weight our fat cells come in contact with many cells that they might otherwise not come in contact with. When these fat cells do contact other cells certain co-factors that are known to start unhealthy cascades are stimulated. In other words it is like a snowball effect that can slowly turn our body in the direction of disease. ASP will increase our storage of fat even when we are already overweight and the last thing we need is more signals to store fat. ASP becomes elevated after we eat and is found to be much higher in people with high body fat percents. ASP is increased by elevated levels of insulin as well!. This is one reason why I strive to decrease the <u>levels of insulin as quickly as possible.</u>

C-reactive protein (CRP) is an indication of inflammation in the body and may also reflect what condition our hearts may be in. Obese individuals usually have higher than normal levels of CRP, which also is predictive of the development of diabetes. The loss of weight alone will decrease levels of CRP. Diets where the primary foods that are eaten are made up of unhealthy processed sugar or high glycemic index foods are associated with high levels of

CRP. The few hormones I have just written about were placed in this book not to confuse you, but to help you understand that our bodies are wired in such a way to keep us healthy. It is our job to make it as easy as possible for these hormones and self defense mechanisms to do their job. If you are overweight it is not enough to simply measure our cholesterol levels, fasting sugar levels and the other "Traditional" tests that are looked at yearly. We should strive to eat as healthy as we can and to stay in the best shape we can. We should feel comfortable going to our primary care doctors and expecting them to know the labs that need to be looked at in order to help us get this job done. If they need some help understanding how this should happen or how they can help, you now have this book you can turn to that will help both of you to better understand how to go about this process.

> _POW_: **_MOST OF THE INFLAMMATION PRESENT WITH WEIGHT GAIN ORIGINATES FROM THE ABDOMINAL AREA. DROPPING INCHES IN THE WAIST LINE CAN BE JUST AS IMPORTANT, IF NOT MORE AS THE SCALE DROPPING._**

Allergies to food:

There are two ways to be "allergic" to food when it comes to weight management. One type of allergic reaction is when a person consumes food items such as shellfish or peanuts resulting in airways closing and a visit to the ER. The other is that when they eat a food it starts certain chemical reactions that actually feel good, or they feel a sort of "high" after they eat them. Like a lot of things in this world when it feels good most people want more of it. The problem with this type of desirable high is that it may be a delayed reaction, so it is hard to tell which food made them feel that way after they have spent time eating additional foods. Why is that bad? Why is it bad to feel so darn good? This sort of high usually results in an enlarging abdomen, hips, or inner thighs. As I tell many patients, it's just not worth it, and to remember the motto "Let your desires obey your reason".

Figure 28: Eight foods that represent up to 90% of the true food allergies in this country
• Milk
• Eggs
• Fish
• Crustacean Shellfish
• Peanuts
• Tree Nuts
• Wheat
• Soy

If the physical response is a mixture of good and bad the body launches a defense. This is an inflammatory response and like most others involves water. So the person begins to swell up globally and this leads to an increase in what they see on the scale. Just like anything else that makes you feel good, you will continue to crave those foods. They see the number on the scale go up, but the amount of food they are eating is small and this is distressing. They don't understand that it is the inflammation and resulting water retention causing the gains but depression sets in anyway. There are a lot of people who eat when they are depressed. If you eat a food and it makes you feel really good, it seems like you can't get enough. I realize removing these food items from your eating regimen is easier said than done, but I have a lot of tricks up my sleeve and I tried my best to make "The Ashworth Weigh" programs as simple as possible.

"The Ashworth Weigh™", the name of the programs I use in my practice pretty much spell out what it is you are eating on a daily basis. It does not take long to figure out what you may be allergic to. It's just that people feel that an allergy to a food must always mean that it makes you go into anaphylactic shock and you end up in the hospital. The truth is the foods that you are allergic to may not do that immediately, but given enough time eating too much of them will render you just as ill, if not more ill than the more common allergic reactions. The "allergy" you will end up with may be weight gain and a subsequent heart condition. If the heart attack that ensues is not an allergic reaction (I admit to using the word allergic loosely) I don't know what is. It is just that in this case the reaction is a constellation of disease processes that end up making you unhealthy over the long term!

I do not base "The Ashworth Weigh™" programs on specific food allergies, but I strive to use the healthiest products on the market and I only use one company for my shake supplements, and that is because the company truly seems to care about what they put out to the consumer. This company's name is the Robard Corporation. Some of the contents in this book are based on concepts that have been brought to my attention by Robard, and their long term dedication in the treatment of obesity has spanned decades.

A few additional foods I have found patients to be allergic to over the years include barley beef, chocolate, citrus, coffee, rye, sugar, tea, and tomatoes. Remember when I use the word "allergic" I am referring not only to the lip and throat swelling more commonly associated with "being allergic to", but also an inability to control how much of a given food that you eat. It goes without saying then that it is vital that I thoroughly investigate every patient's history of food reactions. In keeping with attempting to manufacture the healthiest products possible Robard's shakes are produced without Aspartame which some individuals have been found to be allergic to. You will be hard pressed to find shakes on the market, manufactured for weight management that does not contain this artificial sweetener. In addition to this, Robard has no products that contain fish or shellfish ingredients. The key here as stated numerous times in this book, is that as long as you have had the disorder diagnosed that led to your difficulty in reducing weight the time that you will be required to stay on a weight management program should be the shortest you have ever experienced.

CHAPTER 13

Tell the Truth; Are you Calorie Dense or Nutrient Dense?

The total calories or energy in a given food depends on how many carbohydrates (and types of course), proteins, fat, and alcohol a certain food contains. A **"calorie dense"** food is one that has many calories, but few nutrients. As you can read from what I write in this book about fat and alcohol, the foods containing those types of calories are "calorie dense" foods. Foods that contain large amounts of sugar also fall into this category, which is sometimes referred to as "empty calories". Examples are candies, certain jellies, honey and syrups etc.

"Nutrient Dense" foods provide more nutrition for a relatively small amount of calories eaten. Fruits and vegetables, whole grain breads, and cereals are examples of "nutrient dense" food items. I normally never say that a calorie is just a calorie during weight management. This is because there are so many factors that come into play in terms of how calories are utilized by the body when a person is restricting their calorie intake. When you are done dropping weight and enter the maintenance phase you are not so sensitive to every food item you ingest. It is during this phase, which by the way is a lifelong phase, that a calorie is truly a calorie. When I write this what I am trying to impart is that hopefully during the weight reduction phase you have learned how to eat healthy and have fully adopted this new eating style. So I will take it for granted that each person is eating relatively healthy and what needs to be looked at is the amount of calories you are taking in each day. Sometimes people begin to think because they are eating so healthy they really do not need to watch every calorie they take in. But know this, if a calorie is taken in whether it is a protein, carbohydrate, or fat and it is not used as an energy source it will be converted to fat and stored. There is no pill, injection, or drink that will keep the weight off without using the muscles we are covered from head to toe in.

The take home point to this small section is simple. Eat more nutrient dense foods, but always pay attention to the amount you are taking in. Whether a calorie is nutrient dense or not, a calorie when not used is converted to a fatty acid and stored. The great part about this section on the flip side is that nutrient dense foods will make it easier to exercise. The body has a very hard time turning fat into energy sources. When all you eat is **"calorie dense"** foods, not only is it hard to begin an exercise routine, but it will be even harder to maintain a good cardiovascular pace that will help build endurance and subsequently burn fat.

The muscles prefer to use carbohydrates as an energy source. That is why I am not an advocate for zero or extremely low carbohydrate programs. I prefer to include carbohydrates in my weight management programs, just the right types of carbohydrates. Muscles are much more efficient at converting sugar to energy. Fat is a tough macro-nutrient for the body to convert to a useable form of energy. If muscles have the option to utilize carbohydrates or fat as an energy source the fat will invariably be left alone. Simply put, you fail to lose weight when you eat too many carbohydrates. But there is a caveat to this. What is the favorite type of fuel for the brain? The answer is sugar, glucose or carbohydrates, three words that all pretty much represent the same source of energy. So when professionals come to me for weight management and are physicians, lawyers or pilots, I include a certain amount of carbohydrates. I want them to continue to think clearly so I watch how low I go on the calorie count in general, and give them carbohydrates of the proper type and in the proper amount. So you will not see me advocating cutting out all carbohydrates. There is such a wonderful selection of low glycemic index foods, as well as nutrient dense carbohydrates to choose from.

> _POW: THE MORE NUTRIENT DENSE A NUTRIENT IS THE QUICKER IT WILL MAKE YOU FEEL FULL IN THE FOLLOWING ORDER: PROTEINS, CARBOHYDRATES, AND LASTLY FATS._

TESTIMONIAL:

Deciding to seek medical help for my weight management was an adventure itself. I needed to lose 27 pounds and for 6 years I couldn't lose no matter what diet I tried. Ironically, my insurance would not cover any cost associated with improvement on my health. I begged several of my doctors for assistance with only one of them actually caring enough to help. My general practitioner referred me to Dr. Ashworth in Ormond Beach. With my mind set, I made my appointment determined to finally lose the last bit of weight I had gained from my second child's birth. At first, after receiving my food program menu, I was skeptical if I could really succeed. Once I got started Dr. Ashworth prescribed an appetite suppressant which helped out a lot. I enjoyed the protein drinks, they were very tasty and the variety reminded me of Neapolitan ice cream (and they tasted like them too). The first three days were rough, even with the appetite suppressant medication. I was irritable, short tempered, and the new routine for preparing for each meal was—to me—time consuming and hard. I was used to the fast way of taking care of my hunger. Now I was re-learning how to really take care of what I put in my body and began to change my bad eating habits. The toughest habit to change was eating out of boredom.

I immediately realized that my family ate way too much and I learned that so did I prior to starting this diet. I learned different ways to cook vegetables and pretty much stayed with the pre-sliced/cooked fajita chicken strips (3 oz's = 100 calories) or shrimp for protein to eat every day. My biggest *meal used to be breakfast; I relearned instead to spread out my meals and discovered I was eating 5 times per day. My family even remarked how much I was eating everyday and drinking water like a fish too, but I continued losing weight. It was a testament about not starving me to lose weight. The bathroom soon became my second closest friend due to how much water intake I had. As for the exercise, Dr. Ashworth stressed to me how important the exercise was for 30 minutes a day. I immediately became a walker instead of what I used to do for exercise—jogging. My body was used to the jogging and apparently it didn't work for weight management, so I did the vigorous walks on my treadmill. He told me to try and keep my heart rate between 120 and 150 beats per minute. Since my machine read calories, I evened out the walk so I would burn 400 calories (making my walks 32 minutes). I knew every treadmill was different with the calories burned; however, I only went with mine. I walked every day and on the days I cheated (during Christmas) I calculated the amount of caloric intake and walked longer to burn off the extra food. The weight seemed to come off with no problem.*

I did everything my doctor told me to do and it worked. After the first week of taking my appetite suppressants, I simply used them when I needed them or when I knew I was going to have a long day (hunger would be an issue). My cravings for the junk food soon left after the first week and once in a while I would have a craving (thanks to T.V.). I realized I had to adjust my T.V. watching because of all of the commercials showing you food all of the time. The best part is that once I was near to the amount of weight I wanted to lose, my energy I used to have came back and I did not seem to catch as many colds or the flu like I used to be susceptible to so easily. Since I re-taught myself to limit T.V. time and do something else, I realized I wasn't a couch potato anymore and I completed tasks that needed to be done faster. Now I have a lot more energy to play with my kids, get the house work done, feed everyone (including the animals), and work—everyday.

This used to be very stressful for me, but with my returned energy this wasn't a problem anymore. I discovered what made my weight management so successful (besides doing what the doctor said) was re-programming myself. I programmed myself to eat healthy, fresh vegetables and fruit, and no longer ate them from a can. I learned how to prepare my fresh foods in many different ways and to include 8—8 ounce glasses of water every day. I learned how little fiber is in foods unless we ate them fresh (and/or included fiber supplements). I learned anyone on a diet has to limit sitting in front of the T.V. because of all of the commercials that focus on food (mostly fast food). Exercise was easy for me and now I include it 5 times per week just because I like it. Accomplishing my weight management goal I actually am happier, healthier, feel a lot better (no more back pain), my energy has returned and I sleep like a champ. I had sleep issues before losing the weight, now I sleep soundly and feel revived when I wake up. Since I re-programmed my body to eat fresh foods, I soon discovered that I had to watch what I ate at restaurants. My body was cleansed from all of the toxins with the weight management and cleaner eating over the past several weeks, and to return to eating deep fried foods . . . . oh, what a shock. Needless to say my body didn't like the deep fried foods and I paid for it by praying to the porcelain god until it was out of my system. Since I programmed my body to eat fresh healthy foods, I realize now I need to continue to treat it well and continue to eat what is best. Going back and forth with good and bad foods my body responded immediately reminding me of my previous diet and weight.

Needless to say, my metabolism has sky rocketed. It was "Normal" in the beginning of the program and now after having Dr. Ashworth re-test my metabolism it has increased and is very fast. If I don't eat enough (work interferes a lot with my intake of food), I lose more weight not meaning to, where before I wouldn't. Now if I exercise, I have to make sure I eat more calories or again I will lose weight, what a great feeling!!

Instead of fighting weight off for all of those years I now focus on enough intake of good food like fruit and vegetables and or fiber bars to maintain my weight. I am grateful that my doctor referred me to you Dr. Ashworth because now I am back to my original weight, my life has changed for the best, and my husband has realized how important it is to be at a healthy weight and is now one of your patients!

Thank You!

A very happy husband and (slender) wife ☺

CHAPTER 14

Do not go Overboard with over
the Counter Diet Pills

Diet pills and FDA warnings:

When asked to list all medications a patient takes, many fail to list homeopathic, herbal, or over the counter diet pills as "medications". This is usually because they did not require a prescription to attain them. Sometimes patients will take weight management or "fat burning" pills in the hope that it will speed things up, not realizing that 3 to 5 pounds (this is termed "a medically significant speed of weight management") is as fast as anyone should lose weight. Also, as of January 8, 2009, the FDA started publishing and updating a press release expanding warnings about tainted weight management pills. The most recent list of tainted pills is as follows:

Figure 29: FDA List

FAT LOSS SLIMMING	2 DAY DIET	3X SLIMMING
JAPAN LINGZHI 24 HR	5X IMELDA PERFECT	POWER
DIET	SLIMMING-	3 DAY DIET
7 DAY HERBAL SLIM	8 FACTOR DIET	7 DAY/NIGHT
999 FITNESS	EXTRIM PLUS	FORMULA
ESSENCE	LIDA DAIDAIHUA	GMP
IMELDA PERFECT	PERFECT SLIM 5X	MIAZI SLIM
SLIM	ROYAL SLIMMING	CAPSULES
PERFECT SLIM	FORMULA	PHYTO SHAPE
PROSLIM PLUS	SLIMTECH	SLIM 3 IN 1
SLIM EXPRESS 360	TRIPLESLIM	SOMOTRIM
SUPERSLIM	STARCAPS	ZHEN DE SHOU
VENOM HYPER DRIVE	SLIM UP	SLIM WAIST LINE
3.0	2X POWERFUL SLIMMING	SLIMINATE
SLIM WAIST FORMULA	SUPER FAT BURNER	SLIM EXPRESS 4
SLIM FAST	TRIM 2 PLUS	IN 1
REDUCE WEIGHT	SLIMMING FORMULA	SUPER SLIMMING
SANA PLUS	SLIM 3 IN 1 SLIM FORMULA	POWERFUL SLIM
WAIST STRENGTH	SLIM 3 IN 1 EXTRA SLIM	PERFECT SLIM UP
FORMULA	FORMULA	SLIM 3 IN 1 M18
SLIM BURN	MIAOZI MEIMIAOQIANZ-	ROYAL DIET
SLIM 3 IN 1 EXTRA	IJIAONANG (no I did	NATURAL MODEL
SLIM WAIST	not have a seizure	MEIZITANG
FORMULA	writing this one)	IMELDA FAT
2 DAY DIET SLIM	JM FAT REDUCER	REDUCER
ADVANCE	EXTRIM PLUS 24 HR	FASTING DIET
MEILI	REBURN	BODY SHAPING
7 DAYS DIET	BODY SLIMMING	3 DAYS FIT
COSMO SLIM	BIOEMAGRICIN	7 DIET

A warning from the FDA:

An FDA analysis found that the" undeclared" active pharmaceutical ingredients in some of these products included the following: sibutramine (a controlled substance), rimonobant (a drug not approved for marketing in the U.S. at the time of this printing), phenytoin (an anti seizure medication), phenolphthalein (a solution used in chemical experiments and a suspected cancer causing agent), and bumetanide (diuretic or "water pill"). It is never a good idea to take diuretics or "water pills" during any weight management program. To the contrary, in order for your body to burn fat you absolutely need to be well hydrated. Some of the amounts of "active" pharmaceutical ingredients in the above list far exceeded the FDA-recommended levels, putting consumers' health at risk. In the course of finishing up the last rewrites the FDA announced it was pulling from the shelves the original version of Hydroxycut. This particular product has sold millions of bottles to unsuspecting people that were hoping for what the commercials promised. To the shame of the medical community some of these commercials had doctors endorsing these pills. Liver abnormalities are what the FDA is citing as the main reason the product is being pulled. At the time of this writing it was associated with 5 deaths. As mentioned above one of the aspects of their initial marketing campaign was having doctors on screen talking about the safety and success of this product. The take home point being, if something seems too good to be true, even if it is endorsed by physicians, it probably is.

These weight management products, some of which are marketed as "dietary supplements," are promoted and sold on various web sites and in some retail stores. Some of the products claim to be natural or to contain only herbal ingredients, but actually contain potentially harmful ingredients not listed on the product labels or in promotional advertisements. These have not been approved by the FDA, are illegal, and may be potentially harmful to unsuspecting consumers. The FDA advises consumers who have used any of these products to stop taking them and consult their healthcare professional immediately. The FDA encourages consumers to seek guidance from a healthcare professional before purchasing weight management products. I would also add that you preferably seek that guidance from those healthcare professionals not on the commercials.

"These tainted weight management products pose a great risk to public health because they contain undeclared ingredients and, in some cases, contain prescription drugs in amounts that greatly exceed their maximum recommended dosages," said Janet Woodcock, M.D., director, Center for Drug Evaluation and Research, FDA. "Consumers have no way of knowing that these products contain powerful drugs that could cause serious health consequences. Therefore, the FDA is taking action to protect the health of the American public".

The FDA has inspected a number of companies associated with the sale of these illegal products and is currently seeking product recalls. Based on the FDA's inspections and the companies' inadequate responses to recall requests, the FDA may take additional enforcement steps, such as issuing warning letters or initiating seizures, injunctions, or criminal charges. The health risks posed by these products can be serious; for example, sibutramine, which was found in many of the products, can cause high blood pressure, seizures, tachycardia (rapid heartbeat), palpitations, heart attack, or stroke. This drug can interact with other medications that patients may be taking and increase their risk of adverse drug events. The safety of sibutramine has not been established in pregnant women and lactating women or in children younger than 16 years of age.

Rimonobant, another ingredient found in these products, was evaluated, but not approved by the FDA for marketing in the U.S. The drug, which is approved in Europe, has been associated with increased risk of depression and suicidal thoughts and has been linked to 5 deaths and 720 adverse reactions in Europe over a two year period. New drugs come out frequently, and people will show up at my clinic wanting them immediately. I will wait until a new medication has been in circulation for three to five years before I recommend them to any of my patients.

Health care professionals and consumers should report serious adverse events (side effects) or product quality problems to the FDA's MedWatch Adverse Event Reporting program either online, by regular mail, fax, or phone.

- Online: www.fda.gov/medwatch/report.htm

- Regular Mail: use postage-paid FDA form 3500 available at: www.fda.gov/medwatch/getforms.htm and mail to Med Watch, 5600 Fishers Lane, Rockville, MD 20852-9787

- Fax: (800)FDA-0178

- Phone: (800) FDA-1088

- Information for consumers can be found at: www.fda.gov/cder/consumerinfo/weight_loss_products.htm

I placed the FDA warning in this book because I meet many people that are now my friends and patients who bought all sorts of pills off of the internet. I was amazed what these unscrupulous companies could sell over the internet with very little oversight by government or medical associations. It was not that long ago when physicians working for internet companies could simply have a person fill out a "medical form", return it by email or fax and the physician could get the consumer just about any medication that person desired. There were no face-to-face meetings and no hand or stethoscope ever touched the person ordering the medications. Sometimes the medications were coming from a completely different country. There were no guarantees that what the person was taking was nothing more than a sugar pill. Even worse, the dosage of these medications was under little if any quality control. The chances of purchasing a pill that was way too strong was higher than anyone wanted to admit. This lesson was learned early for me as I was driven along with my fellow medical student colleagues to a hearing where a physician was in the process of losing his license for working with an internet company that was selling medications with no face-to-face meeting between the doctor and patient. Ordering medications over the internet these days is simply taking your life into your own hands. There are now oversight companies that are offering a type of "Seal of Approval". This is a great start, and I welcome this sort of quality assurance.

From my experience, the other over-the-counter (OTC) products on the market when used alone have only a minimal effect on the person's ability to control their hunger. The problem with OTC products is that the people who fail at these "wonder drugs" begin to feel like they have no self control or that there is something "wrong" with them that is not fixable. "Why can't I react to that drug like those beautiful women on TV?" There have actually been exposé's on the producers of infomercials promoting these products that had participants that were actors who never even used the product. Many of these OTC products may be endorsed by a physician on TV, but that is about as far as the medical investigation goes. Some of the above mentioned exposé's have even revealed that the doctor knew little about the product aside from reading a short abstract on a bit of science behind why it *should* work. Do not forget the premise of this book: "It is not your fault." There may be many reasons **why** it is not your fault. And again in my opinion there is no single over-the-counter "wonder pill" that will by itself get the weight off of a person without that pill being accompanied by a complete weight management program designed around helping that person lose weight. To me that means an entire medical work-up. It would be difficult to get that sort of work-up from simply dialing a 1-800 number and giving away your credit card information.

One might begin to wonder if I believe in any sort of "Fat Burning" supplement at all. Actually I have found one root extract that performs exactly the way I would prefer a fat burner to perform. This particular root extract works within the fat cell itself and is completely non-stimulating. Furthermore it does the job better when the person taking the supplement is doing what they are supposed to be doing. This supplement sort of amplifies the efforts of the person taking it. This extract originates from the roots of a plant that grows in India called Forskolin Choleii. As of 2013 I have released this supplement in 2 forms of delivery, a capsule and an injection. The name of the capsule is ***HSL—Metabolic Accelerator***™, and the name of the injection is ***HSL-Release***™. The injection also contains a novel combination of Methionine, Inositol, and Choline (MIC) which increases metabolism as well as insulin sensitivity. The capsule will be available for purchase on the web at www.

metabolicdr.com. and the injection at selected weight management medicine clinics across the U.S.

The extract actually increases the conversion of triglycerides to fatty acids in our fat cells. It is able to accomplish this by stimulating the release of the available amount of <u>hormone sensitive lipase</u> (HSL) in the fat cell. HSL is the key enzyme in the conversion of triglycerides (the storage form of fat) to fatty acids (the form of fat that we can burn for energy). In the years I have been in practice it has become evident that some people simply burn fat at slower rates than others. This has been the case even after I have went through all of the steps of diagnosing and treating the disorders that may have been preventing them from burning any fat at all. When everything has been tried, and reaching those 3-5 pounds of weight loss per week seemed unreachable, *HSL-Metabolic Accelerator*™ has been the answer. You may have noticed though that I did not say that you "do not have to exercise", or that you "do not have to change the way you are eating". To the contrary, if you want this supplement to do its job the initial stimulation to start burning fat needs to be present before anyone starts to take the supplement.

What does this mean to you? It means that there is no "magic bullet" to help you lose weight as you sleep or sit on the couch. Taking the pills listed above and changing absolutely nothing can just about guarantee that you will be gaining the weight back, if any is lost at all. Sometimes people are naïve and believe that a company would never put something dangerous in a pill and sell it on TV or that they would surely get caught before anyone gets hurt. The reality is that companies do sell dangerous pills and people do get hurt. The FDA depends on us, the medical professionals, to do our best to try and educate our patients.

> *POW: REMEMBER THAT A PRODUCT CAN STATE THAT IT DOES NOT CONTAIN EPHEDRA WHEN IN FACT IT MAY CONTAIN "EPHEDRA ALKALOIDS" SUCH AS "BITTER ORANGE" AND "COUNTRY MALLOW".*

CHAPTER 15

Is it Safe to use Appetite Suppressants?

Prescription appetite suppressants:

The disservice doctors have done for our population of overweight patients is giving them a prescription for an appetite suppressant, then giving them a simple diabetic diet (or no diet at all) and telling them to cut back on their eating, exercise more, and return in one month. The problem with this plan is that it is not a plan at all! The problem is that most people actually do stop eating and begin to burn up muscle for nutrients, which drops their metabolism and ends up driving the weight back up once the goal weight is reached, if the goal weight is ever reached at all. This definitely falls under the: "when it's not your fault" category. It is just not as simple as taking a pill or injection and eating less. If it was that simple I don't believe so many people would be overweight. I am not saying I never use appetite suppressants. I just use them as an adjunct to an overall program that looks at the numerous additional issues I bring up in this book.

In my practice I stick to two different appetite suppressant medications: phentermine and diethylproprione (class 4 scheduled substances). A scheduled substance is a medication that is tracked by the Drug Enforcement Agency because of the alleged abusive, addictive nature of the medication. Classes 1, 2, and 3 medications are controlled and tracked more closely. Over the years I have been in practice, both have proven extremely safe just as they have for close to 40 years. The doses I advocate are as follows:

Phentermine: 37.5 mg, one in the morning between 6-8 am. For patients who say they are sensitive to stimulants, we have two options. We can either go with 18.75 mg of phentermine in the morning or diethylproprione 75 mg or 25 mg in the morning.

Diethylproprione: 75 mg, one in the morning between 6-8 am or in combination with phentermine on the same day, but the diethylproprione is taken in the afternoon between 1-3 pm. The diethylproprione is more mild and can be taken later in the day while still allowing the patient to sleep.

The drugs like phentermine and diethylproprione work through an inhibitory effect on the appetite control center of the brain. It has been shown time and time again that these types of medications have very little effect on the levels of serotonin in the central nervous system. I only mention this because I have received a couple of calls from well meaning pharmacists stating that there is a drug interaction between these medications and certain anti-depressant medications that work by increasing the available amount of serotonin in the brain. In all the years I have been in medicine I have yet to see one case of what would be called "Serotonin Syndrome" from the combination of the two medications.

There are many physicians who use a combination of phentermine and Prozac (PhenPro) which started around 1996, which has reported very few side effects. The only problem is that there have been a number of follow-up reports of weight re-gain with the patients that used this combination. I firmly believe this has nothing to do with the medications themselves and would require a more thorough investigation of the program as a whole to determine the cause. A book by the doctor to initially use the combination was written called, Safer than Phen-Fen! In a limited number of patients, I have also used the combination of phentermine and Prozac. The reason for using this combination was because the patient came to my clinic already using Prozac very successfully for depression and required appetite suppression. The two worked well with no side effects to report. Of course, any medication that suppresses the appetite needs to be accompanied by a solid weight management medicine program where any underlying medical causes for weight gain have been investigated.

At the time of this writing, the drug manufacturer Vivus had their weight loss drug Qsymia approved by the FDA's Advisory Panel, as did Arena Pharmaceuticals weight loss drug Belviq. These are the first weight loss drugs approved in thirteen years. Qsymia is a combination of Topamax and Phentermine. The most interesting aspect of this combination is the fact that these two drugs in combination have contradictory instructions as to how to avoid potential side effects. The first precaution that needs to be at the forefront of any female taking this medication is the increased risk of birth defects with Topomax. This becomes more of an issue when one considers the fact that fertility increases with weight loss. In other words as a woman loses weight her chances of becoming pregnant are much better. Phentermine has been around for decades and has a very impressive safety profile. It has the effect of decreasing the appetite therefore decreasing the caloric intake of the individual taking it. Topamax has a couple of interesting instructions for people taking this drug. First, if you take this medicine you should maintain a normal caloric intake! Wait a minute. The desired effect of Phentermine is to make it easier for users to reduce their caloric intake. Secondly, Topamax manufacturers suggest avoiding ketogenic diets. Unfortunately the most popular weight reduction programs on the planet such as the South Beach and Atkins programs advocate reaching a ketogenic state. These weight loss programs actually suggest testing urine samples throughout the program to ensure that the person is producing ketones. In addition, when anyone participates in a reduced carbohydrate program they are essentially on a ketogenic diet! It seems to be counter intuitive to provide warnings such as these and then be marketed as a medication to be used in a weight loss program. The doses at which each of the medications is prescribed when used separately are almost twice as high as the doses they are at when combined in this new drug Qysmia. In addition to this a person could get prescriptions for each of the drugs separately at a cheaper price. So only time will tell.

The other medication making headlines in 2013 is Belviq manufactured by Arena Pharmaceuticals. This is another medication designed to decrease appetite, and make the person feel full sooner after eating smaller amounts of food. The application for approval of Belviq in Europe was withdrawn because of the increased risk of tumors with long term use, psychiatric disorders, and heart valve disorders. This medication works in the same general area of the brain as the medication used in the past referred to as Phen-Fen. That previous Phen-Fen combination included phentermine with fenflouramine and dexfenfluramine, and was suspected as the cause of heart valve abnormalities. Further studies showed that the drug stimulated the <u>serotonin 2B receptors</u>. Belviq primarily stimulates the <u>serotonin 2C receptors</u>. Arena Pharmaceuticals is basing the use of the 2B receptor as opposed to the 2C receptor as the major difference that separates Belviq from Phen-Fen and the cardiac problems that the latter caused. The 2C receptors have failed to show any resulting valvular abnormalities in studies that have lead up to their FDA approval. I still have a "let us wait and see" approach to both of these medications.

We should get one thing straight about the above two appetite suppressants as well as those that I have used. None of these are wonder drugs in and of themselves. Their main job is to take the edge off, to make it easier for you to walk away or push away from the table when you have eaten enough. *When* have you eaten enough? Well, it may be difficult to tell in the beginning of any program. This is why all of the food programs have a specified portion size for every food the person is allowed to eat. Everyone needs to learn to listen to their bodies.

Many people fear that they will be taken off of their appetite suppressants either before they are done reducing weight or when they finish losing their weight. I am not of that camp of thinking: the camp that believes that after 8-12 weeks the patient needs to be taken off their appetite suppressant. These medicines have been around for 40 plus years and have been proven extremely safe. The times when they have caused problems are when they have been attached to other medicines and then used by all medical practitioners, even the ones inexperienced in medical weight management. So, yes, I would much rather have a patient on phentermine during long-term maintenance, much longer than 8-12 weeks. In actuality it feels sort of crazy to even need to justify this issue because it is so full of common sense good medicine. Let us not forget that the two newest drugs being touted as the latest and possibly greatest weight reduction medications approved in the last 13 years, were not only tested on subjects for 1-2 years; but are actually going to be marketed as drugs that can be taken for life! In addition to this one of these new "long-term medications" has phentermine which is still listed as a medication that should be discontinued after 12 weeks. So the next self-proclaimed expert in weight loss that informs you that you need to be taken off of your appetite suppressant because it has been 12 weeks needs to be told to go do their homework and take their head out of the sand.

It is staggering how comfortable so many doctors feel about writing a script for a cholesterol lowering medicine that has shown clear evidence of muscle and liver destroying capabilities; than to write a script for one month's worth of phentermine! Sometimes I get tired of bantering with my colleagues or being at odds with what they consider safe or standard medical protocol. What I strive for in terms of patient care is achieving a healthy performing body that requires fewer useless and/or dangerous medications. All of this will come full circle when the "Standard of Care" undergoes a paradigm shift that focuses on a pro-active approach to health instead of a reactionary one.

POW: APPETITE SUPPRESSION PLAYS A BIG ROLE IN WEIGHT REDUCTION. DO NOT LET AN UNINFORMED DOCTOR TELL YOU HE/SHE IS NOT PERMITTED TO WRITE FOR AN APPETITE SUPPRESSANT, OR THAT YOU NEED TO BE TAKEN OFF IN 12 WEEKS.

CHAPTER 16

Is there anything I can actually eat?

This is where we will look at what foods I approve for my patients to eat. I try to include as many low glycemic index (GI) foods in my programs as possible. In short, this is the section where we talk about macro-nutrients. All of the foods are listed for my patients in their patient packets so that nothing is left to chance. I sort out the number of portions allowed daily, what represents a portion, and how many calories each portion contains. We need to keep in mind how many calories each of the macro-nutrients contain per amount eaten.

The glycemic index (GI) classifies foods according to their potential in raising blood sugar levels, which causes an increase in the body's insulin requirements. Another explanation for the GI is that we are using foods that are digested more slowly. When a food takes longer to make it through the intestines sugar is released into the blood stream slower. Lower spikes in sugar mean lower spikes in insulin. When we are able to avoid higher day-long insulin levels, we avoid <u>increased hunger</u>, high cholesterol, <u>inhibition of fat breakdown</u>, and <u>stimulation of fat storage</u>. With the variety of weight management programs that include solid food, the idea is to include at least one low GI food per meal or to base at least two meals each day on low GI choices.

Carbohydrates:

The buzz word for most of the dieting world is "carbohydrate". Carbohydrates are just one of 4 <u>macronutrients</u>: carbohydrates, fats, proteins and water. Yes, water is a macronutrient. But it remains true that the main source of energy production for most bodily tissues, especially the brain, is carbohydrates. "Glucose" is the fancy word for the form of carbohydrates that are found in the blood, which is simply sugar. Here is the kicker though: any sugar not used for energy by the muscles, brain, or other tissues is stored up as glycogen in those inactive muscles. In the case of the liver, sugar is also converted first to glycogen, and then once the glycogen stores are maxed out in the liver, the glycogen is converted to a fat and stored, hence the diagnosis of fatty liver. These macronutrients aside from water if eaten in excess and not used are converted to fat and stored not just in the liver, but eventually all over the body. Yes everything you eat can be converted to a form of fat and stored!

Simple Carbohydrates:

These are sugars that either occur naturally like fruit sugars, honey, or milk or are processed sugars like corn syrup sugars. Generally, you can find good and bad foods that fall into this category. Some fruits are low on the GI scale and are OK to eat. An apple is better to eat than drinking apple juice, which will spike your sugars. An orange has about the same amount of calories and sugar as a lollipop. But the orange will provide 100% of your recommended daily intake of vitamin C, as well as fiber from the connective tissue in the orange that keeps it together when the outer covering is peeled away. This fibrous nature of an orange or apple is what makes them better than their juice counterparts. The fiber in them helps them to be digested more slowly, thereby avoiding the spike in sugar and subsequent insulin. The fact is we want to be burning excess fat all of the time, not just when we are exercising. We want to burn fat when we are walking to the mailbox or gardening.

Complex Carbohydrates:

Complex carbohydrates are long chains of simple carbohydrates linked together. They are foods known commonly as starches and fibers. These include whole grain wheat bread, long grain brown rice, and wheat pasta, and they provide significant amounts of energy as well as nutrients. The American diet is relatively low in fiber. These complex carbohydrates usually provide more dietary fiber. There are two different types of fiber: water-insoluble and water-soluble. Water-insoluble fiber helps speed passage of food through the digestive track. In other words, this type of fiber will help to pull water into the intestinal track to *relieve constipation*. Just remember there is an "n" in constipation, and an "n" in insoluble fiber. If you are coNstipated reach for the iN-soluble fiber. Water-soluble fiber does the opposite and slows the emptying of food from the intestinal track. These types of water-soluble foods tend to help with hunger a bit, because they stay in your stomach and small intestines longer as they bulk up the stool by soaking up the water around them. These types of fiber would help if a person had diarrhea. My programs always provide plenty of these types of low GI food choices with plenty of the types of fiber the person may need. Everyone is different and the program needs to be tailored to each individual.

Joanne L. Slavin, Ph.D., R.D. published a review article in the periodical "Nutrition" ("Nutrition" 21, (2005) 411-418) that discussed the relationship of fiber intake and body weight. This review provided an update of recent studies of dietary fiber and weight reduction and included weight maintenance. The studies that support dietary fiber intake in the prevention of obesity are strong. Fiber intake is inversely associated with body weight and body fat. The average fiber intake of adults in the U.S. is less than half the recommended levels and is lower still among those who follow an 800-900 calorie low carbohydrate program. Assuring a healthy intake of meat, seafood, fruits and vegetables in any weight management program is the first step. During the maintenance phase, it is important to further increase consumption of low glycemic index fruits, vegetables, whole grains, and legumes.

Each food has been given a GI value. As previously discussed, this value indicates how fast a food is digested and enters the bloodstream as sugar. Regular sugar or white bread has a glycemic index value of 100. The value we strive to be below is 55 in our

<u>choices of fruits, vegetables, and starches.</u> Just remember that song "I can't drive 55". We do not completely restrict everything we eat in an effort to only have foods below 55. Trying to eat like that is just too confining. Below is a list of a few glycemic index values so you can see what types of foods are the best and worst for you to be eating.

Figure 30: LGI Foods	
RICE AND GRAINS:	
Instant rice	87
Whole wheat bread	70
Corn meal	68
VEGETABLES:	
Russet Potatoes 98	
Corn	70
Green peas	51
Black beans	30
Tomatoes	38
DAIRY:	
Condensed milk	61
Yogurt	35
Skim milk	32
Whole milk	27
FRUIT:	
Raisins	65
Mango	55
Banana	60
Kiwi 52	
Orange	40
Apple	40

We always need to find a happy medium. The program you use to lose weight needs to mimic as much as possible how you are going to eat the rest of your life. Even though there are many foods you cannot partake of during a weight management program, this does not mean those same foods have to be completely avoided for a lifetime once in maintenance. You cannot lose weight using a drastic or extremely restrictive program and then expect to be able to keep the weight off after stopping the program. In the maintenance phase there is no way to stay away from every food that has a glycemic index above 55. I cannot stress enough that if there are **medical issues** that have not been addressed and treated, weight maintenance will be impossible, and that is the absolute main purpose for this book. Find out if there are any medical issues that can be addressed then begin the weight management process. The difference between this approach and the years of trying to drop weight that preceded this is that once the weight is lost the medical issue that led to the weight gain will have been fixed, and the yo-yo dieting will be a thing of the past. The injections and lasers and ultra sound devices becoming so prevalent in the medical community do very little in and of themselves to ensure a future that does not include weight re-gain. You can shrink, destroy or cause fat cells to release fatty acids but unless the underlying issue of why that person gains weight so easily is diagnosed all of these devices are very close to useless. I am not writing this simply because it is how I feel. I am writing this because I have witnessed firsthand these devices at work and watched angry, upset, and depressed patients walk out of these clinics. I will admit though that some of these devices have a utility IF they are used in combination with a doctor who has been trained in weight management medicine.

The goal for me has been to make my programs as healthy and easy to follow as possible. Once a person has had their medical issues treated, and their metabolic rate measured they will find weight management easier than they had ever thought. The reason people say weight maintenance is the hardest part is primarily because one cannot be expected to keep weight off when the underlying reasons for the weight gain, like anemia, thyroid problems, or a lack of other vital hormones associated with aging was not addressed. It will also be difficult to maintain weight when they have starved themselves to get the weight off and have managed to burn muscle in addition to the fat. When someone burns muscle they are burning up their metabolic rate, and increasing their "Set Point". This "Set Point" is the weight at which your body always attempts to return to. The major determining factor for a person's set point is the amount of lean muscle tissue their body has. Muscle tissue can represent as much as 40% of a person's metabolism. It is by no means the only determining factor but it truly plays the biggest role when all things are being considered.

Addressing medical issues will always be first on the list in order of importance in getting and keeping weight off. Second on the list is exercise. No one can expect to stay at a normal weight without an effort to get their muscles moving. In maintenance this is the case no matter how little a person eats. If they are not exercising they will slowly begin gaining weight. Yes, I will write that again. If a person is not exercising it does not matter how little they eat, the weight will slowly return. OUCH, I know, this hurts to read. This is because as the amount of food taken in is continually decreased in order to keep from gaining weight, the nutritional intake eventually gets so low that the body begins to burn, yes, you guessed it . . . muscle for nutrients. This eventually drops the metabolism, and the weight starts to sneak back into the hips, abdomen, or where ever they tend to pack it on. As discussed before, the ONLY issue more important than exercise in terms of keeping weight off is making sure that any underlying health issues have been diagnosed and dealt with by a physician trained in weight management medicine. We are living in a society that is technologically growing at a phenomenal rate. We are in no way keeping up genetically or evolutionarily. We still store fat as if we had to hunt and kill our meals. The best we can hope for right now is that nothing is wrong with us medically.

The other macronutrients

The nutrients in the food we eat are important for building and repairing body tissues. One of the main reasons this section on nutrients is in the book is for the person who is having a difficult time finding a weight management medicine physician and has been placed on appetite suppressants. The worse phrase an overweight person can be told by his or her doctor is, "Take this pill and quit eating so much!" Eating and eating correctly is the hallmark of a healthy, rapid weight management program. Nutrients are vital for regulating body processes such as digestion, overall energy production, and muscle contractions while we exercise. I am a big advocate for supplementing a food program with high quality vitamins and minerals. Of course, food is the primary source of energy for our body, so it is important to pay close attention to what you put into your body so you can get as many of the vital nutrients from that food. The old adage stays true: "You are what you eat".

Nutrient and energy requirements for people differ depending on age, gender, body size, physical activity level, metabolic rate, and conditions such as pregnancy. Consequently there is no ideal food plan for everybody, "one size fits all," or cookbook for weight management. What works for one person may not work for the next. That is why my weight management programs are flexible and different for each patient. However, there are standard values that have been put together over the years that have proven to work and meet the dietary needs of most individuals. These standards are referred to as the Dietary Reference Intakes (DRI).

The best way to ensure that you are meeting the (DRI) is to eat a well balanced food program. During weight management it is even more imperative to have a well-balanced food intake. Included in my programs are shake supplements that contain bio-available nutrients. These shakes are used in conjunction with an appropriate combination of low GI fruits, vegetables, and lean meat and seafood's. If you are going to use shakes you need shakes that are manufactured in the appropriate way, which means that during the process of producing them, the nutrients are not de-natured.

A nutrient "de-natured" means the protein or carbohydrate comes unwound and cannot make it into the blood stream during digestion. Or once in the blood the molecule cannot make it into the appropriate cells. This is because the body has specialized cell receptors that are made specifically for such nutrients. When they become unwound they do not fit into that receptor any longer. This will result in a nutrient deficient state that compromises your immune system, among many other problems, and, yes, burns muscle during the process of reducing weight. This in turn will decrease your metabolism and make weight maintenance impossible. When people decide to try some mass produced "All-in-one" shake that promises to burn fat while you sleep, sometimes so much of the de-natured nutrients are left in the gut that water starts to be dumped into the intestines and the result is diarrhea. As a quick quiz what type of fiber would you want if you had diarrhea? You would want to take plenty of soluble fiber.

I have had countless people tell me the Atkins diet did not work for them. When I find out that they were eating 3000 calories of protein, it is no wonder it did not work for them. If you do not burn off the calories you take in, whether they are in the form of carbohydrates, fat, or protein, they will be converted and stored up as fat. Too much of anything, when not handled properly, can be a bad thing. So when these people say they were eating large amounts of steak and eggs and "everything protein," I tell them that sort of diet would not work for anyone when approached in that manner.

> **Figure 31: Macronutrients have the following calorie counts**
> **Protein/Carbohydrate: 4 calories/ gram**
> **Fat: 9 calories/gram**
> **Water: 0 calories/gram**
> **Alcohol: 7 calories/ gram (not a macronutrient but certainly a big part of a lot of people's dietary intake)**

Protein:

Most Americans eat 1 ½-2 times more protein in a day than their body requires. In reality, protein only needs to comprise around 20% of your daily intake if you are a non-athlete. When too much protein is consumed, it is either burned as an inefficient source of energy or converted to fat and stored. In more serious situations, the excess protein, if high enough (usually above 200 grams/day), can cause dehydration and kidney problems. Foods like red meat and dairy products common in the Atkins diet can be high in fat and calories and contribute to the future development of heart disease. Moderation will always be the key, because we definitely need protein in our diet for muscle development and to provide the building blocks for important hormones and digestive enzymes. Protein is needed for a healthy immune system and to carry oxygen on red blood cells, to name just a few.

The basic building blocks of all proteins are **amino acids**. There are two types of amino acids: essential and non-essential. The non-essential is made by the body, and the essential are required to be taken in by the foods we eat. There are nine of those essential amino acids. When we take a look at the foods we eat, we need to try and ensure we are doing our best to supplement ourselves with the correct amount of these amino acid building blocks for those essential proteins. *Complete protein food*s contain all nine amino acids: dairy, eggs, fish, chicken, and red meat. A few incomplete protein foods which lack one or more of the nine essential amino acids are: beans, grains, fruits, nuts, and plant sources of vegetables. The key here is to combine the different foods so that you are taking in enough of the right combinations to make all of the protein you need. As seriously as we may take raising our children, educating ourselves and cultivating our careers; this is the same attitude we need to take in the consumption of the foods we partake of. There is very little in our lives more important than our health. There is very little that has the capacity to have a larger impact on our health status than the types and amounts of food we eat.

Fat:

When trying to understand fat one thing to keep in mind is that fat is a concentrated form of energy. **The body does not like to break down fat and use it for energy (big surprise right?).** When we eat fat we need to also pay attention to the fact that for the same weight of food, for instance one gram of fat versus one gram of another macro-nutrient, there are over twice as many calories in fat as there are in either carbohydrates or protein. Fat has been given a bad rap, but it has a place in our diet. It is unhealthy to attempt to cut out all fats from our diets. Certain vitamins that we absolutely need in order to survive like A, D, E, and K can ONLY be absorbed into our blood stream when they are attached to fatty acids. Fats also contribute to and help develop essential hormones, cellular membranes, and the communication between those cells. From the chapter on bio-identical hormones it is easy to understand how important a well balanced intake of the correct fats can be.

There are good fats and bad fats. The absolute worse fats are the saturated fats. These come primarily from animal sources like high fat red meat and dairy products, and the tasty part of chicken, the skin. These types of fats increase your risk of heart disease dramatically. These types of fats are usually solid at room temperature. A good fat is mono-unsaturated fat (mufa) that has been shown to actually help protect us from heart disease. Research has shown us that in countries that consume a Mediterranean diet high in the use of olive oils or canola oils for cooking the incidence of heart disease is low. Omega-3 fats are a good source of mufa's and are found in canola oil, as well as certain nuts and seeds such as walnuts. Certain fish are also good sources of fat such as Atlantic and Pacific salmon, sea mullet, and southern blue fin tuna. They also generally decrease inflammation in the body which makes weight management easier. Omega-6 fatty acids have also proven to be healthy for the heart and can be found in green leafy vegetables, as well as seeds, nuts, and grains. These types of fats have been known to actually lower total and LDL cholesterol and raise the good HDL cholesterol. The reason HDL is good cholesterol is because HDL attaches to bad cholesterol and carries it back to the liver to be broken down and eliminated. Keep in mind though that a calorie is still a calorie, and when trying to watch how many are taken in, remember that each gram of fat contains 9 calories. It will always hold true that too much of even a good thing can be bad for you.

Water:

Of the three requirements, we'll just call them "The Weight Management Trinity", that I expect from each of my patients on my programs: water, precise nutrition, and exercise, there is only one I ask the patient to try and attempt perfection in, drinking water. The fact is that our bodies are around 70% water, **and muscles are 80% water**. These two reasons alone are usually enough to encourage people to adhere to the water intake required. People will actually lose half the amount of weight they would normally lose in a week if the water is not drank. The water I am referring to is <u>at rest water</u> or water drank when people are not exercising or sweating profusely. People can survive weeks without food, but only days without water. The body's main function with water is temperature regulation. When we exercise all of us need to consistently be taking in water so we do not progress to the level of feeling extremely thirsty. Water will keep us from overheating. This allows us to concentrate on keeping exercise at a level that continues to burn fat. We do this by adjusting one of the three letters in the acronym "FIT": Frequency /Intensity /Time. When at rest the amount of water intake I am referring to is at least 8-8 ounce glasses of water. The water needs to be sipped and drank throughout the day rather than drank in one sitting.

> ### Figure 32: Symptoms of a lack of water
> - Thirst
> - Loss of coordination
> - Muscle cramping
> - Hallucinations
> - Heat exhaustion
> - Heat Stroke

It is not always a lack of potassium that causes muscle cramping. More often than not you should think first of the water intake you have had and if it has been adequate. You may need to drink a rehydration beverage as opposed to grabbing a banana. If you are taking in plenty of water and potassium is the problem, which could be diagnosed by a basic metabolic lab, instead of immediately thinking bananas, know that 4 stalks of celery have more potassium than a large banana. A banana comes with a high glycemic index that will spike your sugar and subsequent insulin levels. Celery on the other hand will exert more energy through digestion than the calories it contains, and does not result in an insulin spike. I realize this may sound amazing but look it up.

When a person is hungry and they know they have just eaten and the hunger is not physiologic, water will help stretch the stomach and signal to the brain that food is not needed. Having a drink of water in between each mouthful of food will help people get full quicker. It is vital though to make sure you are making your way around the plate having a little of all of the food that is nutritious. There is something called the vagal nerve stretch. This vagal nerve wraps around the stomach and when the stomach fills up it will stretch this nerve and signal to the brain it is time to stop eating. One of the important issues is to take your time to eat the meal, at least twenty minutes per meal is the minimum. Water helps the skin stay well hydrated and healthy looking. It will also help to avoid urinary tract infections by keeping the bladder rinsed of stagnant bacteria that can accumulate if one drinks inadequate amounts of water. Drinking a lot of water also keeps the blood thinner, which allows blood vessels to stay clear. There is just a plethora of reasons to drink water.

Alcohol:

Although not a macro-nutrient, enough of the population drinks alcohol that it is worth a mention. If anything is considered an "empty calorie" or a "calorie dense" beverage alcohol falls into that category. It may sound crazy but one of the most common questions I am asked that may actually determine whether a person starts a weight management program is if they will be able to continue to have a couple of alcoholic drinks. I make sure I tell each and every person that I cannot list every food or drink on the food lists because it would be too lengthy. I tell them to contact me by phone or preferably email and ask whether they can have a food or drink they love. Many people forget that I said this and only eat the items on their plan. Those that do forget will return to the clinic complaining of headaches. Headaches are common on a weight management program that has limited the amount of allowable carbohydrates. The headache that results from the withdrawal of both caffeine and carbohydrates can be very severe. Not to mention that a sure way to get a person to quit a program is to take away too many enjoyable activities or foods. Remember moderation is the key in most of what we do in our life. I tell them that they can drink their coffee each day and have a cocktail on the weekend if they choose. If too much of any food or drink occurs the key is to increase the amount of exercise the next day, as opposed to cutting back on the next day's calorie intake. To keep this section short and sweet I figured we would simply list the calorie counts of a few of the more popular drinks so you know how much damage can be inflicted in one night:

Figure 33: Alcohol calories			
•	Beer	12oz	146 calories
•	Pina Colada	4.5oz	262 calories
•	Desert Wine Dry	3.5oz	130 calories
•	Desert Wine Sweet	3.5oz	158 calories
•	Vodka 90 Proof	1.5 oz	110 calories
•	Gin 86 proof	1.5 oz	105 calories
•	Rum 80 Proof	1.5 oz	97 calories

It takes so little of some of these beverages to reach a high calorie intake (1.5 oz = 110 calories) because alcohol is 7 calories per gram. The only other nutrient that beats it is fat itself at 9 calories per gram. One of the major symptoms of being hung over after a night of over drinking is the severe headache. This is experienced by most and is secondary to dehydration. As I have said before what is the one thing that needs to be done perfectly in any weight management program, DRINKING WATER. So not only are you adding empty calories to your intake, you are making it harder for your body to burn off these calories with a lack of water as well. Try to take a sip of water in between each sip of alcohol to minimize the dehydration. Maybe the following morning will not be as miserable or regrettable. Moderation will always be the key. As I have said over the course of this book it is not a good idea to take too many enjoyable behaviors, no matter how hard on weight management, out of a person's life. They just end up getting burned out early and quitting the program. This is the case with alcohol, tobacco, coffee and many others that I have run across.

POW: A CALORIE MAY OR MAY NOT BE CONSIDERED JUST A CALORIE. REMEMBER TO TAKE INTO ACCOUNT HOW MANY CALORIES PER GRAM THE FOOD YOU EAT CONTAINS, AS WELL AS THE TYPE OF CARBOHYDRATES YOU EAT. "I CAN'T DRIVE 55" IS A LITTLE WAY TO REMEMBER TO EAT CARBS THAT HAVE GLYCEMIC INDEXES BELOW 55.

CHAPTER 17

Vitamins: Should I even bother?

Vitamins and Minerals:

Macronutrients are usually eaten in large amounts. Micronutrients in contrast are consumed in small amounts and are represented by vitamins and minerals. Americans spend nearly 2 billion dollars per year on vitamin supplements. The interesting point to note is that vitamins contain no calories at all. Since they have no calories they are unable to provide energy, but they are required for the release of energy in the body. Vitamins also regulate growth and development, metabolism (or fat burning), and a whole array of additional bodily processes.

There are two types of vitamins we need in our body, fat soluble and water soluble. Examples of the fat soluble vitamins are A, D, E, and K and are stored in fatty tissue. These types of vitamins are essential for healthy skin, bones, and blood. The intake of these vitamins need to be monitored because they can accumulate in the tissues and become toxic. Vitamins A and D can damage organs and tissues when taken in excess. The word moderation should come into mind when taking in vitamins also. The exception to the rule is when dealing with D3 which is actually a pro-hormone referred to as cholcalciferol that plays a role in the battle of obesity. Foods rich in D3 are sardines, fortified whole milk, mackerel, and beef liver. D3 also helps with absorption of calcium and strengthens the immune system. Natural sun light is the only biological way (other than buying it in the nutrition store) to synthesize this pro-hormone in the body. The morning sun is the best sunlight and the minimum amount of time to spend in the sun is 20 minutes, with 40% of your body exposed. I usually tell people who get little sun exposure and have a documented lab value that is low is to take 5,000 IU's once per day by mouth.

Water soluble vitamins are vitamins such as the B-Complex vitamins and vitamin C. These vitamins are absorbed in the body's water and are excreted in the urine when taken in excess. This is true at certain amounts, but like anything else if taken in too large an amount even these can cause adverse reactions. These micro-nutrients are essential for energy production, and proper function of the nervous system.

Figure 34: Minerals

1. Examples of **macro-**minerals, need at least 100 mg/day and include:
   - Calcium
   - Phosphorous
   - Magnesium
   - Sulfur
   - Potassium
   - Sodium
   - Chloride
2. Examples of **trace** minerals, need less than 100 mg/day include:
   - Iron
   - Iodide
   - Fluoride
   - Zinc
   - Selenium
   - Copper
   - Chromium (this trace mineral is very effective at helping with insulin sensitivity and sugar cravings)

Minerals are inorganic elements that form most of the hard parts of the body. Some of these include the teeth and bones. Minerals also work in the brain controlling nerves and their conduction. I will give a short list of what I consider some of the more important and then give a brief explanation as to why I think they are so important:

Figure35:	Mineral descriptions
Chromium	Turns food into usable energy, helping insulin prime cells to take up glucose (sugar) out of the blood (remember diabetes)
Potassium	Helps to maintain blood pressure, heart, and kidney function, muscle contraction and digestion (remember exercise and cramping)
B12 & Folate/ Folic Acid	Used in making DNA, the building blocks of genes, helps maintain healthy nerves and red blood production (anemia can result without it)
Magnesium	Triggers more than 300 biochemical reactions in the body and helps to produce energy from the food we eat (energy helps you exercise)
Zinc	Helps keep the immune system healthy and regulates testosterone (can never say enough about testosterone)
Beta Carotene	Converts to Vitamin A, a nutrient essential for healthy vision, immune function and cell growth (important to stay healthy while dieting, if my patients get a serious cold I will raise their calorie count)
Vitamin D3	Works with Calcium to help build and maintain bones (can be dangerous to exercise with osteoporosis) and strengthens the immune system
Vitamin C	Builds collagen, the structural material for bone, skin, blood vessels and other tissue; as well as increases the absorption of iron when taken orally (good for colds, is a strong anti-oxidant)

There are believed to be approximately 20 different minerals that are required for optimal health and the best way to attain them is through a healthy food program. Unfortunately when a person is attempting to lose weight they need to usually lower their calorie intake. At low calorie counts getting the appropriate amount of minerals is difficult when trying to do this just by eating healthy. When trying to lose 15-20 pounds the calorie count is required to be well below the persons resting metabolic rate. This by nature of the calories taken in is impossible to accomplish in a healthy way with food <u>alone</u>. This is when it is extremely helpful to have options for healthy medical shakes that can make up the nutritional deficit. When patients need to lose larger amounts of weight the calorie count need not be so low and in these cases solid food can be eaten in high enough calorie counts to satisfy both the goal of reducing and keeping the program healthy. In my programs I have found that it is extremely motivating for patients to lose 3-5 pounds per week. This is entirely possible to accomplish in a healthy way. I certainly would not have been able to practice **weight management medicine if most of my patients ended up with health problems or weight re-gain** as a by-product of my programs. I have made it my life's goal to create programs that are healthy and motivating in every sense of the word. The programs also need to in some way mimic the way the person will live their lives after the weight management program is finished. As a physician in a town that is small to medium size the only way to survive is to have a successful program that people talk about for years to come. The majority of my patients are referrals from success stories like the ones you read in this book, and from the before and after pictures.

All of the patients understand that I am essentially their personal weight management doctor. They know they can call or email and they will get an answer that day, if not within the hour. If they have some sort of food that is not listed on the food list and they want to know if it is ok to eat I am easy to reach. When seeking a weight management medicine physician this is the type of physician you should strive to see. I have never been the typical doctor and that is how I like it. I went to medical school to practice weight management medicine and I did not waist one minute doing anything else. The first clinic I opened was the first 100% dedicated weight management medicine program in my community.

TESTIMONIAL:

Four years ago, my life was forever changed when a knock on the door in the middle of the night awoke both my husband Paul and I. Only 3 weeks after celebrating a marriage, enjoying the time of our lives was short lived. On the night of November 12, iIn the doorway stood 4 policemen who delivered the news that would change everything forever. A nightmare we hoped would never happen to our family and a pain that is indescribable to bare. Remembering it was like yesterday . . . the policemen delivering the news in my living room, barely containing the stream of tears that rolled down the officers face, bracing himself to tell my husband and I that my dad, Robert F. Grim Sr.; whom I saw hours before having given him a hug and kiss telling him "I love you daddy", was killed while directing a minor traffic incident only minutes away from his office. It would be the last time I would ever see him again, and the last time I would ever know the girl that I once was. His funeral would contain 3 to 4000 law enforcement officials, family and people whose lives he had touched.

The girl, who was known for my devotion to the gym, or often seen roller blading down Granada Boulevard, or perhaps on a run with my dad, was gone. The fun loving, energetic person who loved working out and keeping fit; all of those things that I enjoyed were gone. I no longer enjoyed life and no longer did the things I took pleasure in. I lost that girl I loved and once was. Losing that person also had an effect on my new marriage which also suffered many ups and downs. Not having the desire to live, I also didn't have the love, support and comfort from the man I had intended to spend the rest of my life with. His weakness of infidelity and disrespect would sadly be the demise of our marriage. These hard blows seemed at the time too difficult to bear, and I soon found comfort in food. Someone who always had to watch her weight and be careful of what I would eat soon found herself 30lbs heavier. Someone who typically stayed at 125 to 130lbs found herself weighing in at 160lbs. Not only did I look horrible on the outside, my inside was destroyed also, so I sunk even lower in my addiction to food. I felt like I looked awful and I was buying clothes in sizes I never imagined I would have to buy, and barely squeezing into them.

As I suffered the loss of my dad, along with a husband having done unthinkable things while I grieved over the loss of my dad, I became more depressed. The image I once had of myself and self esteem were gone. But just when I had lost *all hope, thinking I would never feel good internally I became friends with someone whom was already a patient of yours and who was noticeably losing weight and also was feeling better internally herself. When having seen her change in more ways than one, I was given your name. Having seen her results, and becoming herself again I felt I needed the same. Regaining herself worth and self esteem inspired me to see what your office and practice was all about. I was skeptical as I had already tried everything, from the Atkins diet, South Beach Diet, weight watchers, you name it. Even had hired a personal trainer, spending close to $1000.00 but not getting the results I wanted at all. So being someone who is optimistic, I thought what do I have to lose, and so I made my appointment.*

On my initial visit, I not only was inspired but you gave me a sense of hope that I hadn't felt in the last 4 years. I honestly don't think you understand how that felt for me. The affect you had on my life and have had in my life have been the result of your kind words, your efforts to take the time and explain things, to answer questions, to be a coach, to be a friend, to be a doctor, to be understanding to my body type and to taking the time with each of your patients and not rushing them out the door for the next patient. As someone who has worked in the medical field, it was such an amazing feeling that you were so dedicated to your patients and made me want to come back each week. You truly have a gift that gave me that inner strength that has today made me a better person and more importantly a stronger person. Having a sense of self worth and to feel beautiful inside and outside was the medicine I needed.

Since May 2008 I've lost most of the weight I gained over the last 4 years, and I found Tiffany again. It gave me the strength to appreciate and embrace life. It gave me the strength to end a marriage that was toxic in so many ways. The sense of self worth gave me the strength to end a chapter and begin a new one, and I know you always said to me that it was me who did the work, But Dr. Ashworth, it was you who showed me the way and brought me to this happy place in my life. Knowing how this has changed my life, I enjoy seeing you week to week as I am always inspired and always made to feel a way that only empowers me to continue this path. It's such an amazing feeling to know how I was before having met you and knowing the person I am today and all because you helped me believe in myself. You change the lives of others in ways you don't know. You bring happiness to peoples' lives and I hope you know I am forever grateful and how special that makes you. So thank you for helping me see what I lost, because I can now say that I am enjoying life as I have found Tiffany again.

Warmest and Sincerest Regards,

Tiffany

POW: WITH THE HARSH MANUFACTURING AND STORAGE PRACTICES MOST FOODS GO THROUGH ON THEIR WAY TO OUR TABLES, DO NOT IGNORE THE VALUE OF SUPPLEMENTING YOUR INTAKE WITH HIGH QUALITY SUPPLEMENTS.

CHAPTER 18

Do I really have to exercise?

I want everyone to have a better understanding of how calories are handled. The first question to be put out there is what does energy do for us? If I had a nickel for every time I heard someone say "I have absolutely no energy" I could practice weight management medicine for free. In short, energy allows each one of us to move our bodies by muscular contractions.

<u>**Figure 36: Metabolism**</u>

1: In general, "energy" is required for 3 basic functions:

- <u>Basal metabolism - 60-70%</u> (The energy we expend when we are at rest: breathing, our heart pumping blood, controlling bodily temperatures etc.)
- <u>Physical activity for an average person - 15-40%</u> (This is a pretty wide margin! It's a pity that some of us use the same amount of energy devoted to being active that we use to digest the food we eat! We want to strive to be up near the 40% mark when we are calculating the amount of energy expended with physical activity!)
- <u>Digestion - 10-15%</u>

2: Of the above three issues, the one discussed around the water cooler as to why we gain weight so easily is more often than not our Metabolic Rate! So what are some *basic* factors that affect our metabolism?

- Age
- Height
- Weight
- Gender
- Amount of lean muscle (Yes men have more, and yes it usually does mean they can lose weight a bit faster)

When comparing a certain amount or volume of fat and lean muscle, which has the higher metabolic rate? The answer is pretty obvious, muscle is more metabolically active than fat. If this is true then why do so many obese people have a higher metabolic rate than their leaner counter parts? This is because it takes more muscle to walk around with the extra fatty tissue and more muscle to keep the body in an erect position.

Let us take a look at some very basic ways to calculate how many calories you can burn during energy expenditure episodes or during exercise. Physical activity can represent roughly 15% of your total energy expenditure or upwards of 40% of your expenditure. If you feel good and are healthy at a given weight and want a rough estimate and I do mean rough estimate, of how many calories you can take in and maintain that weight there is a rule of thumb calculation one can use. For the calculation you simply take the weight you are presently at and multiply it by 11 (Keep in mind this is a very simplistic way of doing this). By way of example if you weigh 150 pounds and want to stay there the calorie count would be: 150 multiplied by 11 which equal 1650 allowable calories. This calculation automatically assumes the person is undertaking some sort of physical activity four or more days per week. When we simply multiply by the number11 the level of activity would basically be walking your dog as it sniffs and urinates every 10 feet. To top it off, 10 minutes into the walk your 4 year old that begged to go ends up in your arms complaining of leg pain the likes of which no 4 year old on the planet has had to endure. What constitutes easy, moderate, or difficult physical activity is covered further on in the book. To show how easy it is to come close to this calorie count we should calculate the calories of a few foods we might choose to eat in a given day:

Breakfast	Lunch	Dinner
1 Pear: 98 cal	3 oz's Turkey: 132 cal	3 oz's pork chop: 172 cal
1 cup skim milk: 199 cal	Asparagus: 143 cal	1 cup green beans: 44 cal
Yogurt w/ Fruit: 231 cal	2 pcs wheat bread: 130 cal	2 pc's wheat bread: 130 cal
	2 tsp butter: 68 cal	2 tsp butter: 68 cal

The amount of food listed above comes to 1455 calories. This is not a lot of food and does not include any snacks during the day in between the meals, alcohol, soft drinks or deserts. I've written this to show how quickly one can reach a particular calorie count for a day eating healthy. And keep in mind we came up with the limit of 1650 allowable calories per day in a crude and simplistic manner. The above food plan example is very sparse yet it comes surprisingly close to our daily limit. A more accurate method in calculating an allowable daily calorie limit would be to perform a resting metabolic rate, like we administer at the beginning and end of a patient's weight management program. Regardless of how the calories are calculated we will still be surprised how quickly we can arrive at our daily limit.

We can increase the amount of allowable calories in a day by increasing our daily exercise. Exercise physiologists have come up with a number of ways to calculate the amount of calories we burn while performing certain exercises. We need to first understand what an exercise co-factor is. The more strenuous an exercise is the higher the exercise co-factor will be. If we were to perform a brisk walk, a walk that was fast enough that if we went any faster we would need to jog, this exercise would be assigned a co-factor of 1.6. If you multiply this co-factor by our initial allowable daily calories 1650, you arrive at 2600 calories that you could conceivably consume throughout a given day.

Being able to consume 2600 calories without gaining weight has requirements built in. This would require the sort of day where you participated in a daily exercise commensurate with an exercise co-factor of 1.6 or greater. This scenario is one in which we are at a weight we are happy with; where we want to burn as many calories during exercise, as we eat during the day which are above our allowable daily limit. In other words our intake = expenditure.

Calories will end up being used in one of two places. Calories can be used to provide an energy source for physiologic processes such as the movement of our diaphragm as we breathe or the pumping of our heart, or the contraction of our muscles as we exercise. On the other hand, when calories are not burned those calories can end up inside of a fat cell as a <u>storage source</u> contributing to the onset of diabetes. A lot of people tell me they are <u>addicted</u> to food; and as mentioned in this book there is truth to that, but I tell them they are most likely NOT <u>allergic</u> to exercise so get to it!

<u>Figure 37: Co-Factors of common exercises</u>
<u>Very light activities: 1.1</u>
- Simply becoming more active with daily activities of living, weeding the yard, raking leaves (instead of hiring someone else to do it)
- Going from seated to standing multiple times during the day

<u>Light activities: 1.3</u>
- Leisurely Stroll
- Shopping . . Window Shopping
- Walking the dog (Walk does not start till dog has done their business)

<u>Moderate activities: 1.5</u>
- Brisk Walking 15/20 min mile speed (able to talk in a full sentence)

<u>Hard activities: 1.6</u>
- Fast walking (just under a jog)
- Competitive singles tennis

<u>Very hard activities: 1.7</u>
- Stair climbing
- Running
- Jumping rope

Figure 38: Calories burned in 1 hour

Moderately intense activity (1 hour)	Calories burned for 140-150 lb. person	Calories burned for 170-180 lb. person	Moderately intense activity (1 hour)	Calories burned for 140-150 lb. person	Calories burned for 170-180 lb. person
Aerobic Dancing	416-442	501-533	Jumping Rope	640-680	770-820
Backpacking	448-476	539-574	Racquetball	448-476	539-574
Badminton	288-306	347-369	Running (8 mph)	864-918	1,040-1,107
Bicycling (outdoors)	512-544	616-656	Skating (ice or roller)	448-476	539-574
Bicycling (stationary)	448-476	539-574	Skiing (cross-country)	512-544	616-656
Bowling	192-204	231-246	Skiing (downhill)	384-408	462-492
Canoeing	224-238	270-287	Stair Climbing	576-612	693-738
Dancing	288-306	347-369	Swimming	384-408	462-492
Gardening	256-272	308-328	Tennis	448-476	539-574
Golfing (carrying bag)	288-306	347-369	Volleyball	192-204	231-246
Hiking	384-408	462-492	Walking (2 mph)	160-170	193-205
Jogging (5 mph)	512-544	616-656	Walking (3.5 mph)	243-258	293-312

If your weight range is absent from the graph there is an easy way to calculate your calories burned: If you weigh 300 pounds and swim for 1 hour (use the highest number of calories burned in the column containing the highest weight range in the exercise of choice, for swimming that is 492 calories) the calculation would look like: 492 calories multiplied by 300 lbs divided by 175 = <u>843 calories</u> burned in that hour of exercise (roughly).

I have stretches and exercises that will concentrate on loosening up and then strengthening "the core". The core muscle groups are the ones designed to help you stand up straight and keep your balance. The core muscles are mainly in your trunk region like your abdominals and back. When you have the core in good shape it makes working out the remainder of your body easier and less susceptible to injury. Starting off your exercise routine with core based exercises is a great starting point. Even though I may have you simply walking or using an elliptical, there will be a time when you will need to incorporate resistance training (using your own body weight, or using weighted exercises as free weights or in a circuit with machines) to start building lean muscle to keep your metabolic rate in check. These stretches along with full explanations on how to perform them can be found at the end of this book in the appendix section.

When explaining the benefits of exercising while participating in one of my weight management programs I like to keep it simple. Walking is generally considered an easy to perform exercise. It doesn't get much easier in terms of preparation. Just put a good pair of walking shoes on, shorts, a shirt, water bottle, and a way to listen to something and you are ready to go. I have found that listening to music is fine for a while, but within just a few sessions you are back to thinking about how truly boring it is to walk. I tell my patients to go buy books on CD and listen to them instead. It's very difficult to start thinking about your walk when you're trying to follow along to all of the twists and turns in a good mystery. Before the first knife falls in the book you will most likely have finished the walk.

The deal you make with yourself is that you are not allowed to listen to that CD unless you are walking. If I had to choose between walking outside and walking on a treadmill I would pick the treadmill every time. A good treadmill will have a little "give" to the deck as your feet come in contact with it; which is easier on the joints than concrete. If there is foul weather you can still exercise because you have your treadmill. If you have bad knees it is always a good idea to wear a knee brace each time you walk to decrease the wear and tear on the joints, whether the deck is cushioned or not.

The idea is not to simply sweat. I can turn up the temperature in my clinic and get people sweating. Sweating does not mean you are burning calories. I advise my patients to keep their heart rate between 120 and 150 beats per minute. A quick check on your heart rate can be accomplished by taking your pulse for 15 seconds. As long as you are coming up between 30 and 35 beats in 15 seconds you are in a fat burning zone.

TESTIMONIAL:

I had been dieting and exercising for months when I became frustrated because even when I starved myself, I could not get rid of those last 10 lbs. When I realized I wasn't making any progress on my own I decided to look for professional help and found Dr. Ashworth online.

Dr. Ashworth conducted a thorough analysis of my health and my lifestyle habits after which he took time to explain in detail how his weight management program works to increase metabolic rates. With a tailored plan I was able to achieve results in record time. The best part is that after 2 years I have been able to maintain my weight and I look and feel better than ever.

Y J

Orlando, Fl

FIT:

The three things to consider when scrutinizing your exercise routine is the acronym FIT:

Frequency-how many times per week are you doing your exercise.

Intensity-how hard are you working during your walks? You need to be working hard the whole time. This is of course after a proper stretch and 5 minutes of walking slow to warm up the muscles. This time does not count towards your 30 minutes! You need to be cleared by your doctor before starting any exercise program. My patients get all of this in one place obviously.

Time—you need to have your initial goal set for 30 minutes. You may only be able to reach 15 minutes the first 2-3 weeks and that is fine. Of the FIT acronym it will be the Time portion you will be focusing on in the beginning.

Most of us work and have a limited time to dedicate to exercise. Everyone needs to understand that weight management and certainly weight maintenance will be impossible without exercise. If anyone doubts the concept of how important exercise is think of us humans in the pre-historic era! We walked everywhere and had to chase down, kill, or gather our food. The food was always organic and was probably not overeaten. The nature of our existence necessitated retaining a certain amount of lean muscle. Yet even with this exercise, organic foods, and limited supply of this food, we gained weight. Most admittingly, in most cases it may have been a small amount of fat, but we gained nonetheless. This is how we managed to make it through the winters in the cave with 12 other cavemen and women sharing a limited food supply that needed to last through the winter season. We slowly added weight through the spring and summer and burned it slowly through the winter when food became scarce.

Compare the lives we live now to that pre-historic lifestyle. We can drive everywhere. Our food comes to us fully cooked and on a plate or we can simply drive to the supermarket, buy the food and cook it. We usually have jobs that require little if any physical strain or manual labor. If we don't get out and exercise we get very little cardiovascular work, and build little if any lean muscle. This is the perfect environment for the body to store fatty tissue. It's just that the winter never comes. The need to burn the calories off never arrives with this fully automated society we live in. So when you see advertisements for supplements that help you lose weight <u>without exercise or changing anything about your life, change the channel.</u> You are wasting your money in a major way.

If I had to pick one activity that would have the largest impact on our abilities to maintain a normal weight it would be exercise. Yes, not the amount of food we eat, but instead the amount of exercise we get in each day. With a lifestyle that includes exercise, and a body that is without any major health problems the amount of food we eat tends to regulate itself. We start to learn how to listen to our bodies better when we exercise regularly. This includes when we have eaten enough and when we are eating the correct types of food in terms of nutrition.

It is a lot to take in when we begin a fully integrated, life encompassing weight management program. I truly like to keep things simple. Most patients expect to have to join a gym or hire a personal trainer upon beginning the program. I just want my patients to go outside if the weather is nice walk 15 minutes one way, turn around and come back home. I will integrate resistance training (using weights) through the use of circuit equipment or our own body weight as we get closer to our ending goal weight. I am well aware of how important lean muscle is as a contributor to metabolism. I also know that there are other more important issues to pay attention to during the weight management process. When we start the transition phase of increasing our calorie count, we will slowly start to increase our intentions of building more lean muscle. This in turn will allow us to do what we have done and will always need to do, eat food. The big difference of course will be that this will be the **last time** we ever need to lose a significant amount of weight. Why, because we diagnosed the medical problems, addressed any psychological issues, took the time to explain nutrition, and visited each other every week.

We always need to be honest with ourselves. I have found that a food diary is a great way to keep track of what you eat and how often you exercise. When keeping track of what you eat you may find that you do not write down something you would have normally eaten because this time you are going to write it down. Well, write it down any way, be honest with yourself, would you have eaten that cookie? Do not eat it just because you write it down, but mark it down with a star showing that you had the will power to resist the urge to eat it.

Food diaries also give you an idea of what time in each day you get the hungriest. It may be that you get the worst hunger at around 4-6 pm. This is when the phentermine would be wearing off. At this point I could always add a low dose of diethylproprione 25mg (1/3 the dose of the regular pill) at around 1-3pm that will help you through these times of hunger yet still allow you to fall asleep. So I threw the use of an appetite suppressant in there, big deal. If their use was contraindicated in a patient I wouldn't prescribe them. Just another example of when it is nice to have a physician running the weight management program where medications may need to be put on board or taken off.

Another thing to be honest about is how much time you actually exercise. If let's say you were in the pool with the kids for 2 hours. You should not write down that "you were in the pool for 2 hours" when in actuality you only spent maybe 20 minutes doing any strenuous activity completely focused on exercise. When you exaggerate exercise like this you only hurt yourself and your ability to find out which exercises really help you lose weight the best. So write down accurate amounts of food that are eaten and exercise that is performed. I can tell you from personal experience, life is so much easier when exercise is incorporated on a daily basis.

> *POW:* *YOU WILL NEVER BE ABLE TO EAT A LOW ENOUGH AMOUNT OF FOOD WHILE YOU IGNORE EXERCISE AND NOT GAIN WEIGHT. WEIGHT GAIN WITHOUT DAILY EXERCISE IS A GIVEN IN THESE BODIES WE ALL LIVE IN. EXERCISE AND STAY HEALTHY.*

CHAPTER 19

How to Measure Success

Losing the weight is all good, but the <u>real success</u> should be measured by how many patients keep the weight off. I measure the success of my weight management program not by how many people lose the weight or by how many cumulative pounds I can add up over a period of time since I have been in practice, but by how many people are able to keep their weight off over the long term. **The first and most important way to guarantee weight management maintenance is to determine what caused the weight gain in the first place.** Look at some of the celebrities that lose all of the weight only to gain it back. Everyone just takes it for granted that they are getting the best medical care and being tested for all that could be wrong. Chances are they are not being tested for all of the disorders that cause people to have problems with their weight. I think it is safe to assume that they would rather keep the weight off and be healthy. These celebrities then put up with a barrage of condescending comments about their lack of will power and other harmful comments. The goal for me in writing about a few of the more important and prevalent disorders is to teach, not to throw out a bunch of scientific words. The goal is for every obese or overweight person to understand what could be the problem so that they can help their doctors treat them. WHAT did I just say help the doctor? Yes, I did say help the doctor. These men and women are just ordinary people who happened to go through a longer educational process to prepare them to do their chosen profession. As physicians we are certainly not without fault or fallibilities. Although I have found that some of my colleagues may need to be reminded of this fact.

Sometimes a patient just mentioning that they meet some of the symptoms present regarding a certain condition will be enough to spur the doctor into the goal of diagnosing a disorder that has gone unnoticed. I am tired of so many people going undiagnosed as to why they gain weight so easy, lose it so slow and gain it back so quick. I and a few dedicated physicians in this country and abroad, are your advocates for change. My colleagues need to take a moment to look at how happy a person is once they have lost weight and have discontinued ALL of their diabetic or high blood pressure medications. I'm sure they would come to the same conclusion as I have that it makes no sense that they would just eat themselves back into the same diseased state.

So the **real success** will come when doctors begin to accept responsibility for the reasons why their patients are overweight. When that problem is addressed, the treatments for the diabetes or high blood pressure will actually begin to have purpose. We as physicians are supposed to attempt to cure, as opposed to simply keeping a condition "under tight control" like blood pressure or sugar levels. Let's start looking at what caused the patient to have high blood pressure or diabetes. A smart first question for the doctor to consider is did these conditions begin when the weight began to climb. The answer will be obvious. But what is not so obvious is what the doctor decides to do about the overweight condition. Will he or she aggressively treat the obesity or will they continue to write prescriptions for the blood pressure and diabetic medications doing little to nothing about the underlying causes. Is the overweight condition the patient is in being caused by a hormone disorder? If this hormone condition was addressed, and the patient was able to better control their use of calories and lose weight, would the patient even have developed high blood pressure or diabetes? Probably NOT! Or if the doctor treated the diabetic condition with the definitive goal of weight management at the forefront would it make the diabetes treatment more sensible or more effective? With so many of my patients having their high blood pressure or diabetes medicines **stopped** after weight management, the answer is a resounding YES!

I am very honest with my patients. I tell them right from the beginning that their program will not be the easiest or the hardest, but it will be healthy and the most successful. I measure their resting metabolic rate in the beginning and at the end. They will walk out of the transition phase of my program knowing that they have retained all of their muscle, if not having put on more and has had all of their medical needs addressed. For the first time in their lives they will know for a certainty that they have the metabolism to keep the weight off as long as they want to. As a matter of fact, most patients' metabolic rates are faster at the end of the program than when they started. All of those pills out there, that advertise that all you have to do are swallow them and change nothing in your life, are like flushing your money down the toilet. It also wastes your valuable time that could be spent using programs that contain all of the elements of a healthy way to lose weight. The four major parts to look for in a weight management program is a focus on possible medical causes for weight gain outside of eating too much (which may also be a problem), water, exercise, and a healthy way of eating. My programs have these four aspects with emphasis on the first, making sure there is nothing we miss that we can take care of medically that will make the weight management easier and more importantly permanent. I do not want the patient and me banging our heads against the wall as they try to lose weight unsuccessfully because a medical problem was untreated.

To help with hunger and to retain the nutrition so important in a program, we use shakes that are specifically made for weight management programs. I will usually incorporate into my weight management programs 2 to 5 of these 100-160 calorie shakes in combination with solid foods. The goal is to make the weight management program as close to how the person will actually eat after they are done losing the weight. I like to include all of the major food groups with concentration on their effect on the body's insulin response. I do not want someone doing one program to lose weight then having to switch to something completely different once they are done in order to maintain the weight loss.

My goal as a doctor is to treat as many people in my community that have diseases related to being overweight as I can. It is an extremely fun job and there is a lot of satisfaction in what I do. Women and men who lose large amounts of weight and have had their medical problems and or hormones adjusted, if needed, are different people, and I mean that in a positive way. It is not uncommon for them to tell me they cannot remember the last time they felt so good. This is because, as we grow older, the hormone deficiencies creep up on us. It is not like we wake up one morning and say, "Wow, I feel like crap. My hormones must be gone." It's more of an insidious and slow depletion that is hardly noticed. We just get used to feeling like we do and assume it is normal.

It is the same with weight gain, especially weight gain associated with lowering hormone levels. It is a slow process where we gain only ounces per day, ounces that are unnoticed until we go to put a belt on and it no longer fits. Or that summer dress is sticking to just about every part of your body instead of blowing freely in the wind along with your hair. We just need to recognize what is going on and start to do something about it as soon as possible. We need to believe that there just might be something going on beyond just eating too much and not exercising enough. I would never discourage anyone from adding these to their daily activities, but if they keep visiting the scale and it does not seem to be getting lower, then something else may be wrong. The idea is for the person to be able to find a doctor in their community that knows how to adequately treat the obese/overweight patient.

TESTIMONIAL:

Dr. Ashworth,

"Thank you" surely does not seem enough for what you have helped me accomplish. I finally have done it . . . . reached my goal and recognized the person on the inside who has been dying to get out for a lifetime!!!! You have been my mirror. You and I are definitely wired very similar and there were things that you said that really clicked in my head, as well as kicked my ass into gear to just finish what I had started. Why is it we can motivate others so well, and not listen to ourselves??? I saw that in you too as you struggled with exercise and

I appreciated your candidness. Of course, it is only the beginning in many aspects, but now that I have had this glimpse of what my reality is I can move forward and embrace it. I would like to give a big thank you to your staff as well. Each is a unique individual woman with their own strengths and struggles. I wish you continued success in your clinic. I believe in what you are doing and if there is anything I can do to help in the future with a patient or in your clinic just ask.

D M, Florida

As of the writing of this book the above woman had the weight off for over 2 years. The significant part to remember about this weight maintenance is that it reflects the nature of the program in terms of its nutritional value. Not everyone will be able to keep the weight off after losing so much. What I want to emphasize is that it is my responsibility, and I believe every physician out there practicing medicine, to give each man or woman the best chance they can to accomplish what she has: to be able to lose weight not muscle and be able to trust that any underlying medical conditions making weight maintenance difficult are diagnosed and dealt with. Not enough doctors are paying the kind of attention I want them to pay to women like her. I say this because the rates of those that fall under the overweight/obese category seem to continue to rise.

As written earlier in the book this is the first time in history that we have seen young kids being diagnosed with Type II Diabetes Mellitus. This condition used to be called <u>Adult Onset</u> Diabetes. Difficult to call it this when a 15 year old has it, and the reason is a bit more complicated than simply saying it is because the child ate too much and got fat. This may indeed be true, but I certainly do not hear enough physicians trying to make sure they do not have something else going on like growth hormone deficiency or some of the other problems you have read about in this book. It is time for the medical community to wake up and start looking at all of these obese and overweight men, women, and children with a different eye on treatment. We need to look at the patient as a whole, not just a cluster of symptoms that are treated individually. We need to be looking for a possible root cause that may help resolve or at least improve their current disease processes. Admittedly obesity is the root cause for many more diseases, and on the other hand may not be the root cause for some in this book. But this book is going to concentrate on obesity as having the best chance for being the root cause for many of the diseases that plague this country. In other words the person develops a disease like hypothyroidism. This in turn goes untreated because the persons' lab value is borderline low and the doctor is treating the lab and not the person. For the sake of clarity this is called Subclinical Hypothyroidism and the lab values do not necessarily have to be in the abnormal range. The patients' clinical signs and symptoms need to be taken into consideration along with the lab values. In turn the person begins to gain weight, because yes being hypothyroid in most cases leads to weight gain. This extra fatty tissue, especially around the waist leads to the development of diabetes.

So if the doctor would have treated the thyroid condition, the diabetic condition would never have occurred. So the doctor starts to treat the diabetes and continues to ignore the thyroid condition because it fails to fall into the "classic textbook" case for hypothyroidism. Even worse the doctor only ordered a TSH and T4 ignoring the T3 value and fails to make an adequate diagnosis. Why would he or she not order a T3? BIG PHARMA SENDS A GOOD LOOKING PHARMACEUTICAL REPRESENTATIVE WITH A TASTY LUNCH INTO THEIR CLINIC. THIS REPRESENTATIVE PROCEEDS TO TELL THE DOCTOR THAT THERE IS NO NEED TO ORDER THAT SILLY T3 BECAUSE THEIR MEDICATION, CONTAINING ONLY T4 WILL TAKE CARE OF THE CONDITION. AFTER STARING INTO THE EYES OF THAT REP AND WITH A FULL BELLY THE DOCTOR IS SUFFICIENTLY INDOCTRINATED INTO THIS NEW ASCININE WAY OF TREATING, ACTUALLY INADEQUATELY TREATING HYPOTHYROIDISM. I'm not bitter about this, why would anyone think I was bitter or frustrated?

The person continues to gain weight as the doctor adds diabetic medicines that tend to make weight management harder, right along with the untreated thyroid condition. I am witness to these types of scenarios weekly in my practice. If you were to outright ask your doctor to tell you the reasons that people gain weight, the answer may sound something like the following. Here is the official answer given from two M.D.'s—straight out of their published article. It is interesting that the first two reasons given was a nice way of saying that people just eat too much and are basically lazy.

"It is caused by a constellation of factors including excessive energy intake **(EATING TOO MUCH FOOD)**, insufficient energy output **(FAILS TO EXERCISE ENOUGH)**, low resting metabolic rate [RMR]), genetic predisposition, low fat oxidation rate, low sympathetic activity, low plasma leptin level, environment favoring weight gain, psychological stressors and lower socioeconomic status". Bolded statements were added by author of this book for clarity.

In my humble opinion the above physicians were basically saying you eat too much, do not exercise, have a low metabolic rate which may or may not be genetic, cannot process calories in the right way (boy that narrows it down), your nervous system is on the downside which hey, might be the adrenals, you have low leptin levels the hormone that makes you feel full (already proven to be untrue, because for the most part we are actually leptin resistant), you are stressed out because of where you live and because you have no money. This is the point at which the doctor looks at you, hands you a 1200 calorie diet, says appetite suppressants are too dangerous to use and says go lose weight or you're going to have a heart attack.

It was also stated that if a person falls within the overweight range they are still not candidates for any medications to aid in the weight management process, like appetite suppressants. But if they do fall into this category (BMI>24.9) and/or have a BMI greater than 27 **and** also have two disease processes caused by being overweight, they *may be* candidates for medications like diethylproprione or phentermine. So, in order to take medications that are 40 plus years old and have a proven safety record, aside from being overweight, you need to still get just a little sicker before you are eligible for what will most likely be subpar weight management treatment anyway. Oh, and just as you are about to get a handle on your weight management they will discontinue the appetite suppressant because it is for short term use only you silly goose. But since you were not able to get all of the weight off and still are diabetic and hypertensive they will write for 2-3 more medications you are expected to stay on for a life time! Get used to it, people, because this is the standard of therapy for most of the medical community. I don't really care how loud the medical community yells because of what I write.

I have a problem basing my care on how sick a person has to become. I would much rather keep them from getting to the BMI of 27, developing high blood pressure and diabetes. This means I would be practicing medicine in a more proactive manner. Prevention medicine, proactive medicine, metabolic medicine, name it what you will but a paradigm shift is needed and this is what I am talking about in this book. But in order to treat or to prevent, we cannot base treatment on whether a person has developed the disease we are trying to prevent. That does not make a whole lot of sense.

POW: NEVER GAUGE THE SUCCESS OF A GIVEN WEIGHT MANAGEMENT PROGRAM SOLELY ON THE SUCCESS OF PEOPLE LOSING WEIGHT. INSTEAD, GAUGE SUCCESS ON AMOUNT OF PEOPLE THAT HAVE KEPT THEIR WEIGHT OFF.

CHAPTER 20

How to put it all together

Trying to put all of this information together is the catch is it not? This is a lot of information I've given you and it may feel a bit overwhelming. The key is being patient in finding the right people to help you get the job done. Now of course the first step is finding the right doctor. Do not let anyone convince you that there is an easier way to get this job done. If there was then they would already be using it. The epidemic would be slowing instead of gaining momentum. If the doctor you have does not want to embark on this journey with you then find one who will. I have included a lot of information, and have tried to present it in a way that will allow you to understand what may be getting in your way. But I will stress again this is a program that needs to be led by a physician.

Above all else remember that four components need to be present in a program. The program must stress the importance of drinking enough water daily. The program should give you specific options for food selections that are low on the glycemic index scale. The program should stress over and over again how important exercise is to getting and keeping the weight off. Most importantly the program needs to be medically based. There are absolutely too many disease processes out there causing people to gain weight. I will go as far as to say that if you find a weight management program that fails to include a hormonal aspect of medicine, that program is doing more harm than good.

Treating obesity medically will always be the key! It is the secret if there ever was one! Using just exercise or just eating right or even combining the two in just the right way will not work!!! These need to be part of a bigger picture that includes looking at a person's laboratory results, how they feel, how they look, their age and anything else the doctor can think of that will help this person get to the bottom of the medical mystery of why they gain weight and **take the blame off of the patient's shoulders! Because the Weight Gain Is Not Your Fault!**

BONUS MATERIAL APPENDIX A

A weight management medicine program

In this section of the appendix I provide examples of what I include in my own weight management medicine programs. Remember, with any weight management program the initial goal is to find out if there is anything that will get in your way medically. The first order of business as I bring a patient into my program is to measure their Resting Metabolic Rate. If it is low to start with then I know we are off on a fact finding mission to figure out why. The labs that I have listed at the beginning of the book are the ones I commonly order. There are others that I will order if I feel that something out of the ordinary is going on. Since I am commonly considered the "last ditch effort" by many of the people who come to see me there is usually *something* out of the ordinary going on.

Why order an EKG? This is only weight management, right? Wrong, this is weight management medicine and the EKG is important to be able to look for any electrical blocks that may have been caused by an enlarging heart. When a person stays overweight for many years, the heart may get so big it has a hard time delivering enough oxygen enriched blood to itself and small parts of it begin to function poorly. It is simple physics in many respects. As the body gets larger the heart muscle has to also get larger in an effort to pump more blood. Unfortunately the heart can only get so big and can only pump so much blood. The effect of this is that the portion of the heart that is deficient in an adequate blood flow may also experience inadequate electrical flow. Since it is this electrical flow that causes the heart to contract, this will sometimes manifest itself as a portion of heart muscle that does not beat or squeeze blood out of the heart chambers as strongly or efficiently. Medically this is referred to as Obesity Related Cardiomyopathy. When this is combined with high cholesterol, diabetes, and high blood pressure these disorders can take a heavy toll on the heart and congestive heart failure can begin to occur. This is the reason for all of those warnings a person reads when they join a fitness center or hire a personal trainer that usually reads "Make sure your doctor clears you before starting any kind of exercise program". This is yet another reason to be monitored by a doctor. Why just get cleared for exercise by a doctor. Let the doctor handle the entire process from start to finish!

I will then perform a full physical exam, again looking for anything that may make weight management more difficult or dangerous. I listen to the heart for what are called murmurs. These are usually benign and are caused by the valves in your heart not functioning perfectly. Thank goodness perfection is not always needed in many situations, and this just happens to be one of them. However there are murmurs such as Mitral Valve Prolapse that would prohibit a doctor from giving you appetite suppressants. If you have blood pressures that are out of control and consistently elevated, this is another reason when appetite suppressants should not be taken. Getting appetite suppressants off of the internet or borrowing them from a friend can be dangerous as you can see. Not because they may not be what they say they are, which may also be a problem, but from the effect they can have if you have a condition that has gone unnoticed. What I plan on doing is giving you an example of a program that I offer my patients. This is a program that will yield 3-5 pounds of weight management per week in those patients that do their best to stay on top of their responsibilities to the program and more importantly to themselves.

Figure 39: Very low calorie program side effects

- Fatigue: You're consuming fewer calories and what is the best way for your body to battle back and conserve that fat it considers so precious? Keep you on the couch and away from the treadmill. All you can do is drink all of the water, get plenty of rest and do the exercises regardless. In other words PUSH THROUGH IT!

- Dizziness: At times this is because you are drinking so much water and salting so little of what you eat that you end up with low sodium in the blood. The blood essentially gets diluted. The trick is not to cut back on the water, but salt a few of the foods that you eat and the dizziness should resolve in 1-2 days. This should be done under the guidance of a doctor, especially if you have cardiac or high blood pressure issues.

- Headache: This is most likely a carbohydrate withdrawal headache. Especially if you were once a carbohydrate junkie. Just take some ibuprofen for 2-3 days and it will resolve. If you were a caffeine addict as well, whether it is by way of coffee or soft drinks the combination of these two in lesser amounts can make you feel like you're having a stroke. I will not tell my patients to discontinue their intake of coffee if they were the type that had a few cups in the AM. I will however have them slowly decrease the amount of sugary soft drinks.

- Food Cravings: These are not real food cravings if you are getting all of the nutrients you need. Make sure to tell the doctor what it is you are craving so something can be done about it.

- Dry Skin, Brittle Nails, and Hair Loss: When on a truly low calorie healthy program your body will divert energy to the more important bodily functions. It will ignore the ancillary things like nail growth. The slowing down of hair growth or hair loss can be taken care of with Biotin in proper doses and with methionine and Inositol. It is not necessary that you know exactly how much of these supplements to take or how they work. It is your doctors' responsibility to know how to treat you.

- Constipation: This is a condition that can be avoided with plenty of water and twice per day of in-soluble fiber intake. If more drastic measures need to be taken then they can be taken and still will be in the over the counter category most of the time.

Figure 40: Example of a typical 1000 calorie 3 shakes/ day program with solid food	
• 8 glasses of water (8 oz. ea.)	
• 3 Medical Shakes (300 calories total)	
• 2 Lean meat/Seafood (480 calories total)	
• 2 Fruits (180 calories)	
• 4 Vegetables (100 calories)	
• 2 Teaspoons or Capsules of Flaxseed Oil	
Breakfast	1 Shake
Lunch	1 Serving 3-4 oz's Lean Meat/Seafood 1 Fruit, 2 Vegetables
Mid-Afternoon Snack	1 Shake, 1 Fruit
Dinner	1 Shake ½ hr before meal or as a snack later if hungry: 1 Serving 3-4 oz's Lean Meat/Seafood 2 Vegetables
Throughout Day	64 oz's Water Intake

The different aspects of the program in figure 40 above have been put together with many objectives in mind. One is in conjunction with the patient's health status, age, height as well as a few other parameters that when taken together can render a very close estimation of their resting metabolic rate. I always pay strict attention to how the foods taken in will affect each person's insulin levels whether they are a diabetic or not. The biochemistry of different foods has a large implication on what sort of foods I have a patient eat. The shakes above are made for medically supervised programs. That is an incredibly important point by itself. Meaning when you drink these shakes the macronutrients, micronutrients, vitamins, and minerals will make it into your bloodstream. The types of solid foods that are supposed to be used in the food program are low glycemic index foods. I tell my patients if it isn't on the list I give them do not eat it without emailing or talking to me first! Before they leave I ask them one last time what the only part of this program is that they have to do perfectly? Hopefully they answer correctly and say water.

Just like most weight management programs or exercise programs the first two weeks is usually the toughest. Most people already know this and I try my best to give them everything I can to help them get through those first couple of weeks. I will include appetite suppressants if they are not contraindicated and that will usually help quite a bit. One point I want to drive home regarding appetite suppressants is that they do not increase your metabolic rate. They do have a stimulant affect which may make you feel as though you have more energy, but this is temporary and short lived. Increasing metabolism is not an easy task. The primary method for accomplishing this goal is through exercise that builds lean muscle tissue. This type of metabolic increase is more long term because it is derived from muscle tissue. In an otherwise healthy individual the only other way to increase a person's metabolism would be to affect the way fat cells handle the fat that is stored within. Then the question becomes how do I increase the rate of fatty acid formation? Since the storage form of fat is called triglycerides, the question can become even more focused to ask how to increase the rate of conversion of those triglycerides to fatty acids? The answer is that one would need to find a way to increase or stimulate increased activity of a hormone sensitive enzyme that facilitates this conversion. Research has uncovered the answer to this question and named this enzyme Hormone Sensitive Lipase (HSL).

The fact is that people burn fat at different rates. In other words all of us have metabolic rates that are individual to our body, some faster than others. When a person desires to lose weight faster and has had their medical issues taken care of in the entirety, these are the instances when we may intervene and increase the activity of HSL. This also is a temporary measure to be undertaken while the person is building lean muscle that will eventually render the weight management permanent. A root extract out of India holds the answer for increasing the activity of HSL. This all natural extract is called Forskolin Cohleii and the primary delivery method is by taking the capsules orally twice per day. I have literally hundreds of patients that have experienced an additional drop in their weight when they were sure their body was at a plateau it could not recover from. Since discovering this root extract for my patients I had a compounding pharmacy encapsulate the powder for oral consumption. Within ten days of starting the capsules which I named HSL-Accelerator™, the weight management would pick up again or speed up if it had slowed. Of all of the gimmicks out there on the market this is the only compound I have found that truly affects a person's ability to burn fat.

The second week is hard, but for different reasons that are evolutionary in origin. The body goes into a sort of starvation mode and feels as though you must have run out of food and the most important issue is conserving fat. No matter how much pleading I do I usually cannot convince a few of my patients that it is truly a bad idea to hop on the scale every day. So they weigh themselves every day the second week and no matter how hard they bust their butt the weight just stays the same. The body is incredibly efficient at holding onto stored fatty tissue. If they were carrying a baby and traversing some frozen tundra this would be a good thing. This is why I call the second week "The Evolutionary Second Week Slowdown". But because they have weighed themselves every day they get discouraged and do or eat something that sabotages their program. If they really go off the deep end they convince themselves that it must be the program or their body or some other unreasonable conclusion and simply quit. This second week sort of makes up for the large drop most people experience during the first week. Even with this early slow down patients' still experience 3-5 pounds per week when the four weeks are averaged.

TESTIMONIAL:

Dear Dr. Ashworth,

First of all thank you for helping my husband lose so much weight. When he started, at home, he weighed 234 pounds and this morning he weighed 195 pounds! We really appreciate all you have done and will continue to as we try to reach the goal of 180 pounds. We have been telling other people who we know that would benefit from seeing you to come to your clinic for help with their weight. They are seeing that he has been able to lose the weight and his blood pressure medicine has been cut to one third of what it had been after having his open heart surgery. He is able to walk 15 minutes per day, which he was unable to do before losing the weight.

We will stay with you all the way because we know that the Lord has placed you in our lives. We continue to pray God's blessings upon you, your family and office staff! We are looking forward to reading the book when it comes out. Thank you again for all that you have done for us.

Sincerely, R &E

P.S. Thank You for being a friend!

In the above patient I did not need to go extremely low on their calorie count. I simply used two shakes per day at 1500 calories and the weight dropped. Having a Resting Metabolic Rate Analyzer is a big help in deciding what calorie count to go with. Another big issue is how healthy the patient is and if they are going to be able to exercise at all. The above patient had a laundry list of daily medications. The patient suffered from congestive heart failure (CHF), diabetes, high blood pressure, high cholesterol and a couple of more issues that made it hard for him to walk to the mailbox, let alone a half hour per day. We just started slow and worked our way up, eventually walking 15 minutes per day and feeling great.

If a persons' heart is failing then the first thing on the agenda as far as I am concerned is assuring the heart has less tissue to pump to. In congestive heart failure the amount of blood the person can pump out efficiently becomes less and less. In addition, having high blood pressures to pump against does not help either. Patients like the one in the testimonial above are what I live for and one of the many reasons why I am in medical weight management.

The shakes that are listed in Figure: 40 are a vital component to the success of this program. Not just any shake will do. There are a plentiful amount of shakes that claim to be made specifically for reducing weight. The most important issue to be addressed is if the macro-nutrients, micro-nutrients, vitamins, and minerals listed on the label are still intact once these nutrients enter the small intestines. There is a problem with the amount of available protein in a number of shakes currently on the market. If a shake undergoes harsh manufacturing practices it may become denatured, and these proteins WILL NOT make it into your blood stream. If they are not in your blood stream then they are not able to do their job, prevent you from burning up muscle. They essentially become "unwound" and do not fit into the receptors specifically made for them by the body. It gets sort of like trying to fit a square peg into a round hole. If the manufacturing process is too harsh on those fragile nutrients they simply get passed during digestion.

In some instances more than half of a patient's allowable daily calories are from these shakes. With a very low calorie count the body is sure to start breaking down lean muscle to get the protein it needs if all of the nutrition is not present in the form of a combination of these shakes and solid foods. Of course burning up muscle is not the situation I want my patients in. One of the best shake supplement companies I have purchased from and used for years is the shakes offered by Robard Nutrition. As of the writing of this book they make a powdered shake that is mixed with 8-10 oz's of water that is unbeatable in the level of nutrition and patient satisfaction. It comes in a variety of flavors to include vanilla, strawberry, chocolate, and mocha. I love using the shakes because they are perfect for adhering to the old premise, that it is good to eat a number of smaller meals throughout the day. This small intake of nutrients every 2-3 hours allows a steady state level of insulin throughout the day. We want to avoid the high spikes of insulin we get when we have just 2 or 3 larger meals. Having the shakes is an easy, quick way to get your necessary intake of nutrients. Of the three macro-nutrients protein, carbohydrates, and fats the one that gives a person the most satiety, or the feeling of fullness is protein. The shakes I use have 15 grams of protein, and only 2-4 grams of carbohydrates, with 2-3 grams of fat.

When people see what a small amount of food they are allowed to eat they firmly believe they will not be able to do it because of hunger. So lets' reiterate a few items we talked about earlier in the book regarding hunger. What everyone needs to understand is that people get hungry for more than just one reason. One being, the days intake is missing something in your diet that the body requires. The interesting thing about my programs is that I have strived to make sure that all of the nutrient needs are being met at the lowest of calorie counts. This is much easier to accomplish when I have the solid food in combination with the medical shake supplements.

I then take it one step further and make sure that they have retained their lean muscle by taking another resting metabolic rate at the end of the program and compare this to the first. This is actually one of the ways I was able to get referrals from other doctors in the community. They were sure my patient's would quickly gain their weight back with the speed at which I was able to get the weight off. I would then send them the starting and ending metabolic rates and explain why the patient would not be gaining weight back because of anything being done at my clinic. Of course if anyone decides to quit exercising, eating correctly, and ignores all they learned while being at my clinic nothing on this planet can keep them from gaining weight. So once the patient has had their individual medical issues dealt with and have lost their weight; this book's title no longer applies. This is apparent as they walk out of the clinic for the last time with a metabolic rate measurement in hand. Possibly for the first time in their adult lives they will know they indeed have a normal metabolic rate and can keep the weight off for a lifetime.

There is a motto associated with my family crest from the U.K. which reads: "Let your desires obey your reason", and let's just throw in there "do not be quitters!" People come into my clinic and pay me to find out if anything medical is wrong with them, for advice, and the food programs to help them lose weight. Hopefully everyone who reads this book will also find someone to help them diagnose any problems getting in the way and put them on the track to smooth, healthy weight management. The last point I want to make regarding my weight management programs is the transition from a low calorie count using shakes with food, to a calorie count more consistent with the weight they have arrived at when finished with my weight management program. I would like to dedicate some time to explain the importance of this last phase of the weight management process, The Transition.

Transitioning:

What about after the weight is lost—what then? A 6 week transitional period back to food is what happens next. We slowly remove the bulk of the shakes and replace them with foods that the patient enjoys and that are healthy. The idea is to slowly bring the metabolic rate back to where it was before the weight management program began (or, in most cases, higher than what it used to be). As you add more solid food back into the daily eating regimen, the metabolic rate will respond by going up. As you continue to exercise, you will most likely continue to lose weight through this process. Digesting solids requires a bit more energy than liquids and adjusting the metabolism upwards is how your body responds. This leaves a flip side to remember. If the metabolism is coming up as we go back to a normal eating regimen, this means the metabolism was down when we were trying to lose weight. Hard to understand but the truth is that as we decrease our intake our body drops the metabolism in an attempt to spare fatty tissue. I know this when I am calculating how many calories to put a patient on during the active weight reduction phase. Without an appropriate exercise regimen the body will be able to conserve so much energy it would blow most people away! Many try to beat this by continually dropping their intake to lower and lower levels. Once a person reaches critical levels of intake and the diet begins to become non-nutritious the body breaks down muscle. This semi-permanently drops their metabolic rate, and all but guarantees the weight will be gained back. The take home point is always the same, exercise so the weight comes off in a healthy way and stays off over the long term. Never try to force the weight to come off quicker by dropping the daily calories lower and lower.

We take 6 weeks or longer so that we do not assault the digestive tract with a load of solid foods because during the previous 3-4 months a large portion of your daily intake was from liquid shakes. Even if you were on a program that consisted of all food, adding more food needs to be done slowly and smartly. This is a frightening time for a lot of people. They have to go into the transition period with courage and an eye set on a future that includes all that they have hopefully learned throughout the weight management process.

Once we have decided if we are going to include shakes in maintenance and have adjusted the intake to account for this, 2-4 weeks after finishing the transition we will retake the resting metabolic rate. Each patient walks out of the clinic knowing that they have their life in their own hands and finally have some control over what they weigh and how they look. This is because the resting metabolic rate will tell them what their calorie intake should be at the new weight! Right there, in color, will be a representation of how many calories they are able to eat. They will also walk out with a food program put together as a team by myself and the patient that will include as many of the healthful foods the patient likes in their daily menu. This may include continuing to have a couple of shakes or nutritional bars each day.

When I talk about continuing to use the shakes or bars, it is because of studies regarding stimuli narrowing during weight management or maintenance. The less variety of food a person is exposed to, the fewer choices that person will need to make about what they are going to eat each day. Therefore, they will probably fair better on losing or maintaining their weight. Maintenance is the only time when I recommend weighing yourself every day. Graph it by 1 pound intervals so you can see trends early of weight gain, if they are occurring. Do not let things go too long. Get control of whatever it is that is causing the weight gain and fix it as fast as possible.

It has been proven time and again that the people that keep the weight off the longest are the ones that keep a food journal. I would suggest just having a small section in your regular daily journal, if you keep one, where you log in what you had that day to eat. In weight maintenance, there may be some serious emotional adjustments that need to be made to ensure success in keeping the weight off. Try your best to stick to more of a routine eating program. This will hopefully reduce past "food cues" that triggered overeating. I always tell my patients when the choice arises to cheat just repeat the words, "It isn't worth it!" Think about all the hard work it took to lose the weight. It isn't worth it, and that is a fact.

You have the strength inside you to get the job done and stay at your healthy weight. A lot of my patients return every 60-90 days just to check in and see what their weight is on my scale. They want to compare what it is now, as compared to when they left, and see what their body fat percentage is at present. This is also a good time to sit down with the doctor and talk about how things are going. If they are in a trend of gaining weight, it might be time to start on a short 2 week program to jump-start their weight management or to simply get off 5 or 10 pounds quickly and get back on track.

Here is another possibly shocking bit of advice: never declare some type of food completely forbidden. Those types of foods are the ones that used to get you into trouble. But you are a different person after all of the hard work. The food should NOT be one that is eaten weekly, but maybe once per month. In the past, it may have represented a weakness, now it is going to represent your strength! Do not test your resolve too often; there is no reason to do this. Remember the motto, **"Let Your Desires Obey Your Reason"**. These foods are a treat that tastes good, and it will not be a reward related to anything that you have accomplished that day. We never want to reward ourselves with food for anything we accomplish.

Remember, you are really never completely "done". This is a lifetime pursuit of staying fit and eating healthy. This world we live in is sort of like an infection that is not conducive to a healthy lifestyle! It will always be working against you to revert to old easier habits. I will not lie and say that once you reach your goals, it all of a sudden gets easy to stay fit and control all of the facets of your life. My patients will be the first ones to tell everyone about my weaknesses. I don't try to hide them and act impenetrable to cravings or hunger or setbacks in my exercise. I will also tell them that of the three things that we spoke about in the beginning, water, exercise and sticking to an eating program I try to *only let one go.* Maintenance is not hard! Not when the way you lost weight was healthy and you do not stop exercising and drinking water. Reducing weight is the hard part. Once you are done, you need to look back at how hard you worked to do the program correctly. You do not want to go through that again!

Remember we have <u>water, the food we eat, and the exercise we perform</u>. If you falter during maintenance, only let 1 of the 3 falter. Try never to let those 64 ounces of water go! Water is your life line back to where you want to be. For me, it will usually be exercise because of my hectic life. If my exercise falters, I put myself on one of my programs. If I want to go back to eating normal and healthy and at the calorie count I like, then I need to get off my lazy butt and exercise! I will have many "self talks" throughout the day. As I said before, just like you should not be too hard on yourself, I try not to be too hard on myself during these talks. I will usually call someone that I know will show up if I invite them to exercise with me. Besides, I can only take so much abuse from my patients as they gloat about how much better they are doing on their exercise than me. It is never long before I am back to my routine. Like most of you, I become sort of a basket case without regular exercise. The longer I go without it, the harder it is to start back and the more depressed I become. It is a simple fact that exercises makes us feel good!

BONUS MATERIAL APPENDIX B

Stretching

#1: Static Bench:

Directions: Begin by lying on your back with your feet up on a chair or bench. Your body position should be as close to 90/90 degrees as possible. Breath as normal as possible. Relax, holding this position for at least 5-10 minutes. By doing this stretch, you will allow the muscles to release from contractions that are interfering with motor patterns.

#2: Static Extension :

Directions: Kneel on chair or stool, with your hands shoulder width apart and in front of you. Keep your elbows locked straight and move your hips 3-4 inches in front of your knees. Allow your low back to arch with the movement initiating from the tilt of your pelvis. Your shoulder blades should come together and elbows remained locked. Now drop your head and hold the position for 3 minutes. If the low back begins to hurt, back yourself up a few inches towards your knees. This exercise promotes lumbar and thoracic extension through bilateral demand on those areas.

#3: Trunk Rotation/Hip Crossover Stretch:

Directions: Lie down on back with one leg crossed over the opposing thigh. With arms out to the side and palms facing down, lower the raised foot to floor and rotate head to opposite side. It is important to constantly apply pressure to the crossed over leg on top, pushing the knee away from you. Hold this for one minute then repeat with other side.

#4: Prone Cobra:

Directions: Lie face down with your arms at your side. As you inhale, raise your chest off of the ground while simultaneously squeezing your shoulder blades together and rotating your arms so that your palms face away from your body, and your thumbs facing the ceiling.

#5: Super Prone Cobra:

Directions: This movement is the same as the other except as you lift your head; you lift your legs also.

#6: Independent Rotation:

Directions: Begin by lying on your side with a pillow or foam roller under your head. Your legs should be at a 90/90 position with a cushion (A Biocushion if you have one) between your thighs to provide proper spinal alignment. Clasp both hands together and begin to draw one arm up and away as you rotate your torso and allow the involved arm to passively reach the floor. Complete 10 repetitions then on the 11th hold that position for 1 minute. This exercise will allow your upper torso to work independently from your lower.

#7: Groin Stretch

Directions: Begin in a kneeling position and spread legs as far out as you comfortably can. Lean forward, breath gently as you squeeze your inner thighs into the ground for a count of 30-45 seconds then relax and repeat as necessary. Another good groin stretch is to simply sit back against a wall with the flat of your feet against each other; this is sometimes called a butterfly stretch. You then grab your ankles and push your thighs apart with your elbows.

BONUS MATERIAL APPENDIX C

Resistance Training Routine

I will now list a resistance workout that will allow you to build lean muscle. You should not even think about performing any type of exercise program before you stretch properly and are cleared by your doctor. This routine will help you maintain your weight during weight maintenance as well as help with weight management as you approach the end of the active weight management phase. This is because of an increase in muscle mass and consequently metabolic rate. Exercise also increases the amount of brown fat which helps the body access and burn the gold or white fat. These sorts of muscle building exercises will increase insulin sensitivity, as well as a whole laundry list of other positive benefits! For this routine you do not even need to join a fitness center. I will always strive to make anything I ask my patients do as easy to get done as possible.

Equipment needed include:

- Water Bottle (Of course)
- Bosu
- Swiss Ball
- Height Adjustable Aerobic Step
- Dumbbells 10-15 pounds
- Medicine Ball 6 pounds (females), 12 Pounds (males)

Lower body

(Perform 2-3 SETS / 12-15 REPITITIONS FOR ALL EXERCISES UNLESS OTHERWISE INDICATED)

SWISS BALL WALL SQUATS:

This exercise is great for those of us with a bad back. We will not use any weight on our shoulders, just the weight of our body. You simply place the ball at the level of your low back. You then let the ball roll up your back as you squat down. You squat till your legs are at 90 degrees and then come back to almost a straight stand. The idea is to keep the muscles in a contracted state throughout the exercise. In other words don't lock out your knees.

LUNGE ONTO BOSU & ROTATE WAIST TOWARDS THE LEG THAT STEPPED OUT W/MEDICINE BALL:

The whole idea of lunging onto something that is blown up and twisting is that it increases the intensity of the exercises as it tones your legs, buttocks, abs, and back. That's a lot of body parts you are integrating into a single exercise, and you are building your core. That is a good thing. The way to accomplish this exercise is to stand a couple of feet away from the Bosu and lunge onto it, holding the medicine ball at face level. When you reach the 90 degree bend in your knee turn your whole body to the side that lunged out. When you turn you will be holding the medicine ball out in front of you. As you are coming back up bring the medicine ball back out to the front. Repeat this with the same leg 10-15 times, and then switch legs and the direction you turn. When you are attempting this for the first time it would be a good idea to not use the ball, and even perform the exercise next to a counter you can hold onto for balance purposes.

LEG CURLS W/ SWISS BALL Super Set/w TRICEP KICKBACKS:

This exercise takes quite a bit of core balance. First you lay on your back, on the floor with your feet on the Swiss ball. Using your abdominal, back, and leg muscles lift the lower part of your body off the ground. It is ok to have your arms out at 90 degrees for help with balance. The key to this is that you have to have your buttocks off the floor. Your weight should be held up with your feet on the Swiss ball and your upper back and arms. You then use your ham string muscles (the ones on the back of your legs) to roll the Swiss ball up towards your buttocks as far as you can. You should feel this in your legs and buttocks

Upper Body

(Perform 2-3 SETS / 12-15 REPITITIONS FOR ALL EXERCISES UNLESS OTHERWISE INDICATED)

PUSHUPS (21's, 15'S, OR 9'S) USING AN AEROBIC STEP OR BOSU:

I have three different names for this exercise because how many you can do will depend on how long you've been working this group of exercises. The idea is to perform a regular pushup to the left or right of the step. When you finish each pushup you place the hand closest to step on it and then tap the step with the other hand and repeat. Then you place yourself in front of the step and perform a pushup, when you reach the top of the pushup one hand goes on top of the step then the other joins it, then one comes off and then the other hand does the same. You then move to the right side of the step and repeat as with the left. The idea is to do 7, 5, or 3 reps at each of the positions. <u>An aerobic step is better for this exercise than the Bosu.</u>

SWISS BALL DB CHEST PRESS:

This is a simple exercise where you lay on the Swiss Ball positioning the ball between your shoulder blades. The lower half of your body extends straight out away from the Swiss ball and your legs are bent at 90 degrees, feet flat on the floor. You then begin pushing the dumbbells away from your body alternating each arm. But do not let your arm rest on the Swiss ball as your other arm is pushing the weight up. Do not lock your arms out at the top either, but keep them slightly bent.

SWISS BALL LATERAL FLY'S FOR BACK AND SHOULDERS:

For this exercise you lay with your chest on the Swiss ball keeping your balance with your body extended straight back, legs open as you balance yourself between your toes on the floor and your chest on the ball. You then take the lighter dumbbells and extend them out to the side with your elbows slightly bent. The range of motion is from the floor, just before relaxing and then back to horizontal (as if you were trying to fly). As an alternate you can also sit on the Swiss ball, bend at the waist till chest touches your thighs and perform the same exercise.

SWISS BALL TRICEP KICK BACKS:

For this exercise you stand and then lean over at the waist, placing one hand on the Swiss ball. With the other hand you bring your elbow and upper arm into a 90 degree position and then you straighten out your arm to the rear while holding a light dumbbell. You will be working the back of your arms. When I write super set I mean you do one set of one exercise then go straight to the other with no rest.

BENCH DIPS:

For this exercise you place both of you arms behind you, supporting yourself on a bench or chair situated at your back. Your legs will be extended out in front of you and your feet resting on the Swiss ball. You then bend your arms till they are at 90 degrees, then push yourself back up as you keep your balance with your legs on the Swiss ball. The only way to keep your balance is to tighten your abdominal muscles or your core muscles!

BONUS MATERIAL APPENDIX D

Pool exercises

For the millions of people out there with limited range of motion, and arthritic joints there are always pool exercises. These are specifically designed for those patients with limited exercise capacity. You will most likely find that as the weight is lost the pain in the knee, hip, and low back areas improve somewhat.

- Stand in neck deep water and have your arms at your side. Then raise your arms, keeping them straight and palms facing forward to the surface. Return arms to sides turning your palms over and repeat. Perform 3 sets of 20 repetitions. Rest 1 minute between sets.

- In same position keep arms extended out and move them in small or large circles, whichever feels more comfortable? Perform 3 sets of 20 repetitions. Rest 1 minute between sets.

- Prop your elbows on the side of the pool with your back towards the ledge. Raise left leg upwards in the water, keeping them straight. As left leg is lowering, right leg should be coming up. Perform 3 sets of 20 repetitions. Rest 1 minute between sets.

- For this exercise you will need a kickboard. Grab the kickboard and place it under your forearms, holding the board and extending the arms. Your head and upper shoulders should be above the water. Kick from one end of the pool to the other. Use either the flutter kick or the frog kick. Perform 3 sets of 20 repetitions. Rest 1 minute between sets.

• Stand in chest deep water. <u>Walk </u>in the pool, back and forth lifting your knees as high and close to 90 degrees as possible during the walking. Perform 3 sets of 20 repetitions. Rest 1 minute between sets.

• Stand in chest deep water. <u>Jog </u>in the pool, back and forth except this time you do not need to lift your knees as high during the walking. Just bring them 2-3 inches from the bottom of the pool. Perform 3 sets of 20 repetitions. Rest 1 minute between sets. It's fine to jog in a pool because you only weigh 10% of your weight in the water!

• Stand in chest deep water with left side of body next to the edge of pool holding yourself steady with your left hand. Stick right leg a few inches away from the other leg and begin turning the leg in small circular motions keeping the leg straight. Repeat this except turned the other way and using the other leg. Perform 3 sets of 20 repetitions. Rest 1 minute between sets.

• Stand in neck deep water and have your arms extended straight out just under the surface of the water. Then begin to push your arms out in front of you as if you were clapping. Keep your elbows straight and your palms facing out in front of you with thumbs pointing up. As you begin the backwards stroke turn thumbs down and hand over with palms facing the opposite direction. Perform 3 sets of 20 repetitions. Rest 1 minute between sets.

BONUS MATERIAL APPENDIX E

HSL-Accelerator™

"Accelerate your Metabolic Rate!":

If there has ever been or ever will be what people would consider a "Magic Pill for weight management" this is it! Among the many hormones and enzymes that have been studied through the years Hormone Sensitive Lipase (HSL) is in my opinion the most promising for actually increasing the amount of fat available for the body to either use as an energy source or excrete as a by-product of weight management. Think of HSL as the gate keeper for fat cells. Studies have shown that it is the increased concentration of HSL inside of the fat cell that leads to maximally stimulated release of free fatty acids. HSL has to be stimulated to accomplish this job. The "Accelerator" in HSL-Accelerate, is called Forskolin Cohleii, which is a root extract that has been proven to stimulate increased activity of HSL, thereby accelerating weight management.

Studies have shown that it is the increased concentration of HSL inside of the fat cell that leads to maximally stimulated release of free fatty acids. This simply means that Forskolin increases the activity of HSL which turns the storage form of fat, which are triglycerides into fatty acids! Once these fatty acids are released with the help of HSL-Accelerator™ they are used for energy decreasing the size of fat cells all over the body! Even more exciting is that as you exercise a particular area of the body, taking this compound will allow you to spot reduce that area. More can be found on this compound that I have used to help people lose weight for years at: www.metabolicdr.com.

REFERENCES

Chlebowski, RT. "Influence of Estrogen Plus Progestin on Breast Cancer and Mammography on Postmenapausal Women: The Women's Health Initiative Randomized Trial," The Journal of the American Medical Association, Vol. 289, No. 24, June 25, 2003. (http://jama.ama-assn.org/cgi/content/full/289/24/3243).

Velazquez EM, Mendosa S. Hamer T, Sosa F, Glucck CJ. Metformin therapy in women with polycystic ovary syndrome reduces hyperinsulinenia, insulin resistance, hyperandrogenemia, and systolic blood pressure, while facilitating mestrual regularity and pregnancy. Metabolism 1994, 43: 647655.

SiegelRL, Jermal A, Ward EM. Increase in incidence of colorectal cancer among young men and women in the United States. Cancer Epidemiol Biomarkers Prev. 2009;18(6):1695-8.

Tohme C, Labaki M, Hajj G, Abboud B, Noun R, sarkis R. Colorectal cancer in young patients: presentation, Clinicopathologic characteristics and outcome. J Med Liban. 2008 Oct-Dec;56(4):208-14.

Montalcini T, Gorgone G, Federico D, et al. Association of LDL cholesterol with carotid atherosclerosis in menopausal women affected by the metabolic syndrome. Nutr Metab Cardiovasc Dis. 2005 Oct;15(5):368-72.

LaRosa JC, Women, lipoproteins and cardiovascular disease risk. Can J Cardiol. 1990 May;6 Suppl B:23B-9B.

Kim HK, Kim CH, Kim EH, et al. Impaired fasting glucose and risk of cardiovascular disease in korean men and women: the Korean heart study. Diabetes Care. 2013 Feb;36(2):328-35.

Ford ES, Zhao G, Li C. Pre-diabetes and the risk for cardiovascular disease: a systematic review of the evidence. J Am Coll Cardiol. 2010 Mar 30;55(13):1310-7.

Liu S, Willet WC, Stampfer MJ, et al. A prospective study of dietary glycemic load, carbohydrate intake, and risk of coronary heart disease in US women. Am J Clin Nutr. 2000 June,71(6):1455-61.

Levitsky YS, Pencina MJ, D' Agostino RB, et al. Impact of impaired fasting glucose on cardiovascular disease: the Framingham Heart Study. J Am Coll Cardiol. 2008 Jan 22;51(3):264-70.

Hokanson JE, Austin MA. Plasma triglyceride level is a risk factor for cardiovascular disease independent of high-density lipo protein cholesterol level: a meta-analyses of population-based prospective studies. L Cardiovasc Risk. 1996 Apr;3(2):213-9.

Viles-Gonzales JF, Fuster V, Corti R, Badimon JJ. Emerging importance of HDL cholesterol in developing high risk coronary plaques in acute coronary syndromes. Curr Opin Cardiol. 2003 Jul;18(4):286-94.

Slaminen M, Kuppamaki M, Vahlberg T, Raiha I, Irjala K, Kivela SL. Metabolic syndrome and vascular risk: a 9-year follow-up among the aged in Finland. Acta Diabetol. 2011 Jun;48(2):157-65.

Tanko LB, Bagger YZ, Qin G, Alexandersen P, Larsen PJ, Christiansen C. Enlarged waist combined with elevated triglycerides is a strong predictor of accelerated atherogenesis and related cardiovascular mortality in postmenopausal women. Circulation. 2005 Apr19;111(15):1883-90.

McSweeney JC, Cody M, O'Sullivan P, Elberson K, Moser DK, Garvin BJ. Women's early symptoms of acute myocardial infarction. Circulation. 2003 Nov 5;108921):2619-23.

Akishita M, Hashimoto M, Ohike Y, et al. Association of dehydroepiandrosterone-sulfate levels with endothelial function in postmenopausal women with coronary risk factors. Hypertens Res. 2008 Jan;31(1):69-74.

Sablik Z, Samborska-Sablik A, Goch JH. Concentrations of adrenal steroids and sex hormones in postmenopausal women suffering from coronary artery disease. Pol Merkur Lekarski. 2008 Oct;25(148):326-9.

Slowiaska-Srzednicka J, Malczewska B, Srzednicki M, et al. Hyperinsulinaemia and decreased plasma levels of dehydroepiandrosterone sulfate in premenopausal women with coronary artery disease. J Intern Med. 1995 May;237(5):465-72.

Schufelt C, Bretsky P, Almeida CM et al. DHEA-S levels and cardiovascular disease mortality in postmenopausal women: results from the National Institutes of Health—National Heart, Lung, and Blood Institute (NHLBI)-sponsored Women's Ischemia Syndrome Evaluation (WISE). J Clin Endocrinol Metab. 2010 Nov;95(11):4985-92.

Dandona P, Dindsa S, Chauduri A, Bhatia V, Topiwala S, Mohanty P. Hypogonadotrophic hypogonadism in Type 2 diabetes, obesity and the metabolic syndrome. Curr Mol Med. 2008;8(8):816-28.

Mathus-Vliegen EM; Obesity Management Task Force of the European Association for the Study of Obesity. Prevalence, pathophysiology, health consequences and treatment options of obesity in the elderly: a guideline. Obes Facts. 2012;5(3):460-83.

Zitzman M. Testosterone deficiency, insulin resistance and the metabolic syndrome. [review]. Nat Rev Endocrinol. 2009;5(12):673-81.

Jones TH, Saad F. The effects of testosterone on risk factors, and the mediators of, the atherosclerotic process [review]. Atherosclerosis. 2009;207(2):318-27.

Provel CM, Beulens JW, van der Schouw YT, et al. Metabolic syndrome model definitions predicting type 2 diabetes and cardiovascular disease. Diabetes Care. 2012 Aug 29 [Epub ahead of print].

Kershaw EE, Flier JS, Adipose tissue as an endocrine organ. J Clin Endocrinol Metab. 2004;89(6):2548-2556.

Wang C, Jackson G, Jones TH, et al. Low testosterone associated with obesity and the metabolic syndrome contributes to sexual dysfunction and cardiovascular disease risk in men with type 2 diabetes [review]. Diabetes Care. 2011;34(7):1669-75.

Gooren LJ, Begre HM,. Diagnosing and treating testosterone deficiency in different parts of the world: changes between 2006 and 2010. Aging Male. 2012;15(1):22-27.

Huggins C, Hodges CV. Studies on prostatic cancer: I. The effect of castration, of estrogen and androgen injection on serum phosphatases in metastatic carcinoma of the prostate. Cancer Research. 1941;1:293-297. Reprinted by: J Urol. 2002;167(2 Pt 2):948-51.

Huggins C, Hodges CV, Stevens RE. Studies on prostatic cancer: II. The effects of castration on advanced carcinoma of the prostate gland. Archiv Surg. 1941;43(2):209-23.

Morgentaler A. Goodbye androgen hypothesis, hello saturation model [editorial]. Eur Urol. 2012 Jun 16 [epub ahead of print].

Garcia-Cruz E, Piqueras M, Huguet J, et al. Low testosterone levels are related to poor prognosis factors in men with prostate cancer prior to treatment. BJU Int. 2012 May 15 [Epub ahead of print].

Shin BS, Hwang EC, Im CM, et al. Is a low serum testosterone level a risk factor for prostate cancer? A cohort study of Korean men. Korean J Urol. 2010;51(12):819-23.

Morgentaler A. Low testosterone levels are related to poor prognosis factors in men with prostate cancer prior to treatment. BJU Int. 2012 May 15 [Epub ahead of print].

Khera M, Grober ED, Najari B, et al. Testosterone replacement therapy following radical prostatectomy. J Sex Med. 2009;6(4):1165-1170.

Shabsigh R, Crawford ED, Nehra A, Slawin KM. Testosterone therapy in hypogonadal men and potential prostate cancer risk: a systematic review. Int J Impot Res. 2009;21(1):9-23.

Li Z, Maglione M, Tu W, et al. Meta-analysis: pharmacologic treatment of obesity. Ann Intern Med 2005;142:532-46.

Vetter ML, Faulconbridge LF, Webb VL, Wadden TA. Behavioral and pharmacologic therapies for obesity. Nat Rev Endocrinol 2010;6:578-88.

Hendricks EJ, Greenway FL, Westman EC, Gupta AK. Blood pressure and heart rate effects, weight loss and maintenance during long-term phentermine pharmacotherapy for obesity. Obesity 2011;19:2351-60.

Rosenstock J, Klaff LJ, Schwartz S, et al. Effects of exenatide and lifestyle modification on body weight and glucose tolerance in obese subjects with and without pre-diabetes. Diabetes Care 2010;33;1173-5.

Lijesen GK, Theeuwen I, Assendelft WJ, Van Der Wal G. The effect of human chorionic gonadotropin (HCG) in the treatment of obesity by means of the Simeons therapy: a criteria-based meta-analysis. Br J Clin Pharmacol 1995;40:237-43.

Astrup A, Rossner S, Van Gaal L, et al. Effects of liraglutide in the treatment of obesity: a randomised, double-blind, placebo-controlled study. Lancet 2009;374:1606-16. Erratum in *Lancet* 2010;375:984.

Wood S. Liraglutide in nondiabetics: weight and BP improve at two years in extension trial. October 11, 2010. HeartWire. http://www.theheart.org/article/1132987.do. (Accessed June 10, 2013).

Kaptein EM, Beale E, Chan LS. Thyroid hormone therapy for obesity and nonthyroidal illnesses: a systematic review. J Clin Endocrinol Metab 2009;94:3663-75.

Verrotti A, Scaparrotta A, Agostinelli S, et al. Topiramate-induced weight loss: a review. Epilepsy Res 2011;95:189-99.

Ben-Menachem E, Sander JW, Stefan H, et al. Topiramate monotherapy in the treatment of newly or recently diagnosed epilepsy. Clin Ther 2008;30:1180-95.

Gadde KM, Franciscy DM, Wagner HR, Krishnan KR. Zonisamide for weight loss in obese adults: a randomized controlled trial. JAMA 2003;289:1820-5.

Colman E. FDA Briefing Document. NDA 200063. *Contrave* (Naltrexone 4 mg, 8 mg/Bupropion HCl 90 mg extended release tablet). December 7, 2010. http://www.fda.gov/downloads/advisorycommittees/committeesmeetingmaterials/drugs/_endocrinologicandmetabolicdrugsadvisorycommittee/ucm235671.pdf. (Accessed June 10, 2013).

Orexigen. Our approach to obesity treatment. http://www.orexigen.com/product-candidates.html. (Accessed June 10, 2013).

Anon. FDA declines to approve Orexigen's *Contrave*, requests new trial. February 3, 2011. http://fdanews.com/newsletter/article?articleId=133950&issueId=14435. (Accessed June 10, 2013).

Kopelman P, Groot Gde H, Rissanen A, et al. Weight loss, HbA1c reduction, and tolerability of cetilistat in a randomized, placebo-controlled phase 2 trial in obese diabetics: comparison with orlistat (*Xenical*). Obesity 2010;18:108-15.

Ozcan L, Ergin AS, Lu A, et al. Endoplasmic reticulum stress plays a central role in development of leptin resistance. Cell Metab 2009;9:35-51.

Kang JG, Park CY. Anti-obesity drugs: a review about their effects and safety. Diabetes Metab J 2012;36:13-25.

European Medicines Agency. Withdrawal of the marketing authorisation application for *Belviq* (lorcaserin). May 30, 2013. http://www.ema.europa.eu/docs/en_GB/document_library/Medicine_QA/2013/05/WC500143811.pdf. (Accessed June 4, 2013).

Takeda. Amylin and Takeda discontinue development of pramlintide/metreleptin combination treatment for obesity following commercial reassessment of the program. August 5, 2011. http://www.takeda.com/news/2011/20110805_3889.html. (Accessed June 10, 2013).

FDA. FDA Briefing Document. NDA 22529. May 10, 2012. www.fda.gov/downloads/AdvisoryCommittees/CommitteesMeetingMaterials/Drugs/

EndocrinologicandMetabolicDrugsAdvisoryCommittee/UCM303198.pdf. (Accessed June 10, 2013).

Costantino D, Minozzi G, Minozzi E, Guaraldi C. Metabolic and hormonal effects of myo-inositol in women with polycystic ovary syndrome: a double-blind trial. Eur Rev Med Pharmacol Sci. 2009 Mar-Apr;13(2):105-10.

Raffone E, Rizzo P, Benedetto V. Insulin sensitiser agents alone and in co-treatment with r-FSH for ovulation induction in PCOS women. Gynecol Endocrinol. 2010 Apr;26(4):275-80.

Larner J. D-chiro-inositol—its functional role in insulin action and its deficit in insulin resistance. Int J Exp Diabetes Res. 2002;3(1):47-60.

Larner J, Brautigan DL, Thorner MO. D-chiro-inositol glycans in insulin signaling and insulin resistance. Mol Med. 2010 Nov-Dec;16(11-12):543-52. Epub 2010 Aug 27. Review.

Predicting Development of Proliferative Diabetic Retinopathy. By Kristen Harris Nwanyanwu and colleagues. Diabetes Care 2013, pages 1562-1568

Differences in A1C by race and ethnicity among patients with impaired glucose tolerance in the Diabetes Prevention Program, by W.H. Herman and colleges. Diabetes Care 30: 2453-2457, 2007.

Li Z, Maglione M, Tu W, et al. Meta-analysis: pharmacologic treatment of obesity. Ann Intern Med 2005;142:532-46.

Vetter ML, Faulconbridge LF, Webb VL, Wadden TA. Behavioral and pharmacologic therapies for obesity. Nat Rev Endocrinol 2010;6:578-88.

Hendricks EJ, Greenway FL, Westman EC, Gupta AK. Blood pressure and heart rate effects, weight loss and maintenance during long-term phentermine pharmacotherapy for obesity. Obesity 2011;19:2351-60.

Rosenstock J, Klaff LJ, Schwartz S, et al. Effects of exenatide and lifestyle modification on body weight and glucose tolerance in obese subjects with and without pre-diabetes. Diabetes Care 2010;33;1173-5.

Lijesen GK, Theeuwen I, Assendelft WJ, Van Der Wal G. The effect of human chorionic gonadotropin (HCG) in the treatment of obesity by means of the Simeons therapy: a criteria-based meta-analysis. _Br J Clin Pharmacol_ 1995;40:237-43.

Astrup A, Rossner S, Van Gaal L, et al. Effects of liraglutide in the treatment of obesity: a randomised, double-blind, placebo-controlled study. _Lancet_ 2009;374:1606-16. Erratum in _Lancet_ 2010;375:984.

Wood S. Liraglutide in nondiabetics: weight and BP improve at two years in extension trial. October 11, 2010. _HeartWire._ http://www.theheart.org/article/1132987.do. (Accessed June 10, 2013).

Kaptein EM, Beale E, Chan LS. Thyroid hormone therapy for obesity and nonthyroidal illnesses: a systematic review. _J Clin Endocrinol Metab_ 2009;94:3663-75.

Verrotti A, Scaparrotta A, Agostinelli S, et al. Topiramate-induced weight loss: a review. _Epilepsy Res_ 2011;95:189-99.

Ben-Menachem E, Sander JW, Stefan H, et al. Topiramate monotherapy in the treatment of newly or recently diagnosed epilepsy. _Clin Ther_ 2008;30:1180-95.

Gadde KM, Franciscy DM, Wagner HR, Krishnan KR. Zonisamide for weight loss in obese adults: a randomized controlled trial. _JAMA_ 2003;289:1820-5.

Colman E. FDA Briefing Document. NDA 200063. _Contrave_ (Naltrexone 4 mg, 8 mg/Bupropion HCl 90 mg extended release tablet). December 7, 2010. http://www.fda.gov/downloads/advisorycommittees/committeesmeetingmaterials/drugs/ endocrinologicandmetabolicdrugsadvisorycommittee/ucm235671.pdf. (Accessed June 10, 2013).

Orexigen. Our approach to obesity treatment. http://www.orexigen.com/product-candidates.html. (Accessed June 10, 2013).

Anon. FDA declines to approve Orexigen's *Contrave*, requests new trial. February 3, 2011. http://fdanews.com/newsletter/article?articleId=133950&issueId=14435. (Accessed June 10, 2013).

Kopelman P, Groot Gde H, Rissanen A, et al. Weight loss, HbA1c reduction, and tolerability of cetilistat in a randomized, placebo-controlled phase 2 trial in obese diabetics: comparison with orlistat (*Xenical*). *Obesity* 2010;18:108-15.

Ozcan L, Ergin AS, Lu A, et al. Endoplasmic reticulum stress plays a central role in development of leptin resistance. *Cell Metab* 2009;9:35-51.

Kang JG, Park CY. Anti-obesity drugs: a review about their effects and safety. *Diabetes Metab J* 2012;36:13-25.

European Medicines Agency. Withdrawal of the marketing authorisation application for *Belviq* (lorcaserin). May 30, 2013. http://www.ema.europa.eu/docs/en_GB/document_library/Medicine_QA/2013/05/WC500143811.pdf. (Accessed June 4, 2013).

Takeda. Amylin and Takeda discontinue development of pramlintide/metreleptin combination treatment for obesity following commercial reassessment of the program. August 5, 2011. http://www.takeda.com/news/2011/20110805_3889.html. (Accessed June 10, 2013).

FDA. FDA Briefing Document. NDA 22529. May 10, 2012. http://www.fda.gov/downloads/AdvisoryCommittees/CommitteesMeetingMaterials/Drugs/EndocrinologicandMetabolicDrugsAdvisoryCommittee/UCM303198.pdf. (Accessed June 10, 2013).

Centers for Disease Control and Prevention, Children and diabetes—more information. April 3, 2012. http://www.cdc.gov/diabetes/projects/cda2.htm. (Accessed June 7, 2012).

American Diabetes Association. Type 2 diabetes in children and adolescents. *Diabetes Care* 2000;23:381-9.

American Diabetes Association. Standards of medical care in diabetes—2012. *Diabetes Care* 2012;35(Suppl1):S11-S63.

Canadian Diabetes Association. Canadian Diabetes Association 2008 clinical practice guidelines for the prevention and management of diabetes in children. *Can J Diab* 2008;32(Suppl 1):S1-S201.

International Expert Committee. International expert committee report on the role of the A1C assay in the diagnosis of diabetes. *Diabetes Care* 2009;32:1327-34.

Sellers EA, Moore K, Dean H. Clinical management of type 2 diabetes in indigenous youth. *Pediatr Clin North Am* 2009;56:1441-59.

Today study group. A clinical trial to maintain glycemic control in youth with type 2 diabetes. *N Engl J Med* 2012;366:2247-56.

Katz LE, Magge SN, Hernandez MI, et al. Glycemic control in youth with type 2 diabetes declines as early as two years after diagnosis. *J Pediatr* 2011;158:106-11.

Barnes NS, White PC, Hutchinson MR. Time to failure of oral therapy in children with type 2 diabetes: a single center retrospective chart review. *Pediatr Diabetes* 2012. Published on-line ahead of print, May 31, 2012. Doi: 10.1111/j.1399-5448.2012.00873.x.

Copeland KC, Becker D, Gottschalk M, Hale D. Type 2 diabetes in children and adolescents: risk factors, diagnosis, and treatment. *Clin Diabetes* 2005;23:181-5.

Jacobson-Dickman E, Levitsky L. Oral agents in managing diabetes mellitus in children and adolescents. *Pediatr Clin N Am* 2005;52:1689-1703.

Flint A, Arslanian S. Treatment of type 2 diabetes in youth. _Diabetes Care_ 2011;34(suppl 2):S177-S83.

Benavides A, Striet J, Germak J, Nahata MC. Efficacy and safety of hypoglycemic drugs in children with type 2 diabetes mellitus. _Pharmacotherapy_ 2005;25:803-9.

Li XJ, Yu YX, Liu CQ, et al. Metformin vs. thiazolidinediones for treatment of clinical, hormonal, and metabolic characteristics of polycystic ovary syndrome: a meta-analysis. _Clin Endocrinol_ 2011;74:332-39.

Balen A, Homburg R, Franks S. Defining polycystic ovary syndrome. New criteria say that hyperandrogenism and ovarian dysfunction are needed. _BMJ_ 2009;338:a2968.

Franks S. When should an insulin sensitizing agent be used in the treatment of polycystic ovary syndrome? _Clin Endocrinol (Oxf)_ 2011;74:148-51.

Diamanti-Kandarakis E, Economou F, Palimeri S, Christakou C. Metformin in polycystic ovary syndrome. _Ann N Y Acad Sci_ 2010;1205:192-98.

Katsiki N, Hatzitolios AI. Insulin-sensitizing agents in the treatment of polycystic ovary syndrome: an update. _Curr Opin Obstet Gynecol_ 2010;22:466-76.

Tang T, Lord JM, Norman RJ, et al. Insulin-sensitising drugs (metformin, rosiglitazone, pioglitazone, D-chiro-inositol) for women with polycystic ovary syndrome, oligoamenorrhoea and subfertility. _Cochrane Database Syst Rev_ 2010;(1):CD003053.

Ortega-Gonzalez C, Luna S, Hernandez L, et al. Response of serum androgens and insulin resistance to metformin and pioglitazone in obese, insulin-resistant women with polycystic ovary syndrome. _J Clin Endocrinol Metab_ 2005;90:1360-65.

Glueck CJ, Moreira A, Goldenberg N, et al. Pioglitazone and metformin in obese women with polycystic ovary syndrome not optimally responsive to metformin. *Hum Reprod* 2003;18:1618-25.

Glintborg D, Andersen M. Thiazolidinedione treatment in PCOS— an update. *Gynecol Endocrinol* 2010;26:791-803.

Gharib H, Tuttle M, Baskin HK, et al. Subclinical thyroid dysfunction: a joint statement on management from the American Association of Clinical Endocrinologists, the American Thyroid Association, and the Endocrine Society. *J Clin Endocrinol Metab* 2005;90:581-5.

U.S. Preventive Services Task Force. Screening for thyroid disease. *Ann Intern Med* 2004;140:125-7.

Baskin HJ, Cobin RH, Duick DS, et al. American Association for Clinical Endocrinologists medical guidelines for clinical practice for the evaluation and treatment of hyperthyroidism and hypothyroidism. *Endocr Pract* 2002;8:457-69.

Razvi S, Weaver JU, Butler TJ, Pearce SH. Levothyroxine treatment of subclinical hypothyroidism, fatal and nonfatal cardiovascular events, and mortality. *Arch Intern Med* 2012;doi:10.1001/archinternmed.2012.1159.

Rugge B, Balshem H, Sehgal R, et al. Screening and treatment of subclinical hypothyroidism and hyperthyroidism. Comparative Effectiveness Review No. 24. *AHRQ Publication No. 11(12)-EHC033-EF*. Rockville, MD: Agency for Healthcare Research and Quality. October 2011.

Danzi S, Klein I. Subclinical hypothyroidism and the heart: the beat goes on. *Thyroid* 2012;22:235-6.

Traub-Weidinger T, Graf S, Beheshti M, et al. Coronary vasoreactivity in subjects with thyroid autoimmunity and subclinical hypothyroidism before and after supplementation with thyroxine. *Thyroid* 2012;22:245-51.

Bahn Chair RS, Burch HB, Cooper DS, et al. Hyperthyroidism and other causes of thyrotoxicosis: management guidelines of the American Thyroid Association and American Association of Clinical Endocrinologists. *Thyroid* 2011;21:593-46.

Collet T, Gussekloo J, Bauer DC, et al. Subclinical hyperthyroidism and the risk of coronary heart disease and mortality. *Arch Intern Med* 2012;10.1001/archinternmed.2012.402.

North American Menopause Society. Menopause practice; a clinician's guide. Section G. Hormonal drugs. October 2007 (Edition 3). http://www.menopause.org/Portals/0/Content/PDF/G.pdf. (Accessed April 12, 2012).

Electronic Orange Book. Approved products with therapeutic equivalence evaluation. Current through February 2012. http://www.fda.gov/cder/ob/. (Accessed April 12, 2012).

Drugs@FDA. http://www.accessdata.fda.gov/scripts/cder/drugsatfda/. (Accessed April 12, 2012).

PL Detail-Document, Bioidentical Hormones. *Pharmacist's Letter/Prescriber's Letter.* October 2003.

Boothby L, Doering PL, Kipersztok S. Bioidentical hormone therapy: a review. *Menopause* 2004;11:356-67.

Health Canada. Drug product database online query. http://webprod.hc-sc.gc.ca/dpd-bdpp/index-eng.jsp. (Accessed April 12, 2012).

Anawalt BD. Guidelines for testosterone therapy for men: how to avoid a mad (t)ea party by getting personal. *J Clin Endocrinol Metab* 2010;95:2614-7.

Coplan B, Spiegel J, Bleaman I, Roch J. Testosterone replacement therapy: take an informed, individualized approach. *JAAPA* 2011;24:42-7.

Wang C, Nieschlag E, Swerdloff RS, et al. ISA, ISSAM, EAU, EAA and ASA recommendations: investigation, treatment and monitoring of late-onset hypogonadism in males. *Aging Male* 2009;12:5-12.

Bhasin S, Cunningham GR, Hayes FJ, et al. Testosterone therapy in men with androgen deficiency syndromes: an Endocrine Society clinical practice guideline. *J Clin Endocrinol Metab* 2010;95:2536-59.

Liverman CT, Blazer DG. Testosterone and Aging: Clinical Research Directions (2004). Institute of Medicine / Board on Health Sciences Policy. http://www.nap.edu/books/0309090636/html/. (Accessed June 9, 2010).

Wu FC, Tajar A, Beynon J, et al. Identification of late-onset hypogonadism in middle-aged and elderly men. *N Engl J Med* 2010;363:123-35.

Cook NL, Romashkan S. Why do we need a trial on the effects of testosterone therapy in older men? *Clin Pharmacol Ther* 2011;89:29-31.

Anawalt BD. Male hypogonadism. January 2010. Merck Manual. http://www.merckmanuals.com/professional/sec17/ch227/ch227b.html. (Accessed February 13, 2011).

AACE Hypogonadism Taskforce. American Association of Clinical Endocrinologists Medical Guidelines for clinical practice for the evaluation and treatment of hypogonadism in adult male patients-2002 update. *Endocr Pract* 2002;8:440-56.

Harman SM. Testosterone in older men after the Institute of Medicine Report: where do we go from here? *Climacteric* 2005;8:124-35.

The Practice Committee of the American Society for Reproductive Medicine. Treatment of androgen deficiency in the aging male. *Fertil Steril* 2006;86:S236-40.

Kuzmarov IW. An overview of testosterone deficiency and hypogonadism. *Geriatr Aging* 2008;11:S4-S9.

Srinivas-Shankar U, Roberts SA, Connolly MJ, et al. Effects of testosterone on muscle strength, physical function, body composition, and quality of life in intermediate-frail and frail elderly men: a randomized, double-blind, placebo-controlled study. *J Clin Endocrinol Metab* 2010;95:639-50.

Emmelot-Vonkk MH, Verhaar HJ, Nakhai Pour HR, et al. Effect of testosterone supplementation on functional mobility, cognition, and other parameters in older men: a randomized controlled trial. *JAMA* 2008;299:39-52.

McLachlan RI. Certainly more guidelines than rules. *J Clin Endocrinol Metab* 2010;95:2610-3.

Fernandez-Balsells MM, Murad MH, Lane M, et al. Adverse effects of testosterone therapy in adult men: a systematic review and meta-analysis. *J Clin Endocrinol Metab* 2010;95:2560-75.

Bhasin S. The brave new world of function promoting anabolic therapies: testosterone and frailty. *J Clin Endocrinol Metab* 2010;95:509-11.

Basaria S, Coviello AD, Travison TG, et al. Adverse events associated with testosterone administration. *N Engl J Med* 2010;363:109-22.

Cunningham GR, Toma SM. Clinical review: Why is androgen replacement in males controversial? *J Clin Endocrinol Metab* 2011;96:38-52.

Folia C, Bain J. Options in testosterone therapy. *Geriatr Aging* 2008;11:S19-S26.

Omega-3 fatty acids: an update. *Pharmacist's Letter/Prescriber's Letter* 2007;23(8):230807.

U.S. Canola Association. I. Essential fatty acids and fat nomenclature. http://www.uscanola.com/index. asp?type=B_BASIC&SEC={1F7232BD-72B3-42CD-86E7-2C11E3942C6D}&DE={BBB69F6A-98A3-4388-96A7-2EAEFC063C4E}. (Accessed May 10, 2010).

Jellin JM, Gregory PJ, et al. *Natural Medicines Comprehensive Database*. http://www.naturaldatabase.com. (Accessed May 10, 2010).

Harris WS, Mozaffarian D, Rimm E, et al. Omega-6 fatty acids and risk for cardiovascular disease: a science advisory from the America Heart Association Nutrition Subcommittee of the Council on Nutrition, Physical Activity, and Metabolism; Council on Cardiovascular Nursing; and Council on Epidemiology and Prevention. *Circulation* 2009;119:902-7.

American Heart Association. New release. Healthy vegetable oils associated with reduced heart attack risk, lower blood pressure. http://americanheart.mediaroom.com/index. php?s=43&item=459. (Accessed May 10, 2010).

Ferrara LA, Raimondi AS, d'Episcopo L, et al. Olive oil and reduced need for antihypertensive medications. *Arch Intern Med* 2000;160:837-42.

Fernandez-Jarne E, Martinez-Losa E, Prado-Santamaria M, et al. Risk of first non-fatal myocardial infarction negatively associated with olive oil consumption: a case-control study in Spain. *Int J Epidemiol* 2002;31:474-80.

Brackett RE. Letter Responding to Health Claim Petition dated August 28, 2003: Monounsaturated Fatty Acids from Olive Oil and Coronary Heart Disease. *CFSAN/Office of Nutritional Products, Labeling and Dietary Supplements*. 2004 Nov 1; Docket No 2003Q-0559. Available at: http://www.fda.gov/

ohrms/dockets/dailys/04/nov04/110404/03q-0559-ans0001-01-vol9.pdf. (Accessed May 13, 2010).

Livieri C, Novazi F, Lorini R. [The use of highly purified glucomannan-based fibers in childhood obesity]. Pediatr Med Chir 1992;14:195-8.

Walsh DE, Yaghoubian V, Behforooz A. Effect of glucomannan on obese patients: a clinical study. Int J Obes 1984;8:289-93.

Cairella M, Marchini GAD. [Evaluation of the action of glucomannan on metabolic parameters and on the sensation of satiation in overweight and obese patients]. [Article in Italian] Clin Ter 1995;146:269-74.

Heymsfield SB, Allison DB, Vasselli JR, et al. Garcinia cambogia (hydroxycitric acid) as a potential antiobesity agent: a randomized controlled trial. JAMA 1998;280:1596-600.

Muller WE, Singer A, Wonnemann M, et al. Hyperforin represents the neurotransmitter reuptake inhibiting constituent of hypericum extract. Pharmacopsychiatry 1998;31:16-21.

Cangiano C, Ceci F, Cancino A, et al. Eating behavior and adherence to dietary prescriptions in obese adult subjects treated with 5-hydroxytryptophan. Am J Clin Nutr 1992;56:863-7.

Vahedi K, Domingo V, Amarenco P, Bousser MG. Ischemic stroke in a sportsman who consumed MaHuang extract and creatine monohydrate for bodybuilding. J Neurol Neurosurg Psychiatr 2000;68:112-3.

Doyle H, Kargin M. Herbal stimulant containing ephedrine has also caused psychosis. BMJ 1996;313:756.

FDA Takes Aim at Ephedra. The Washington Post. Available at: www.washingtonpost.com/wp-dyn/articles/A33439-2000Mar17.html (Accessed 19 March 2000).

Lee NA, Reasner CA. Beneficial effect of chromium supplementation on serum triglyceride levels in NIDDM. Diabetes Care 1994;17:1449-52.

Penzak SR, Jann MW, Cold JA, et al. Seville (sour) orange juice: synephrine content and cardiovascular effects in normotensive adults. J Clin Pharmacol 2001;41:1059-63.

Smedman A, Vessby B. Conjugated linoleic acid supplementation in humans—metabolic effects. Lipids 2001;36:773-81.

Health Canada requests recall of certain products containing ephedra/ephedrine. Health Canada Online 2002. www.hc-sc.gc.ca/english/protection/warnings/2002/2002_01e.htm (Accessed 9 January 2002).

Bravata DM, Sanders L, Huang J, et al. Efficacy and safety of low-carbohydrate diets: a systematic review. JAMA 2003;289:1837-50.

Atkins RC, Ornish D, Wadden T. Low-carb, low-fat diet gurus face off. Interview by Joan Stephenson. JAMA 2003;289:1767-8, 1773.

Foster GD, Wyatt HR, Hill JO, et al. A randomized trial of a low-carbohydrate diet for obesity. N Engl J Med 2003;348:2082-90.

Ludwig DS. The glycemic index: physiological mechanisms relating to obesity, diabetes, and cardiovascular disease. JAMA 2002;287:2414-23.

Foster-Powell K, Holt SH, Brand-Miller JC. International table of glycemic index and glycemic load values: 2002. Am J Clin Nutr 2002;76:5-56.

Nykamp DL, Fackih MN, Compton AL. Possible association of acute lateral-wall myocardial infarction and bitter orange supplement. Ann Pharmacother 2004;38:812-6.